My Secrets of Natural Beauty

My Secrets of Natural Beauty

by
Virginia Castleton Thomas

Keats Publishing, Inc. New Canaan, Connecticut

Copyright © 1972 by Virginia Castleton Thomas

All Rights Reserved

Published in 1972 by Keats Publishing, Inc.
212 Elm Street, New Canaan, Connecticut 06840

ISBN 0-87983-019-1

Library of Congress Catalog Card Number: 72-76464

Printed in The United States of America

To my beloved Richard, who taught me that beauty of self and soul is our birthright.

Author's Foreword

Ever since woman's reflection was caught in still water or the polished surface of the first mirror in ancient China, her vanity and her desire to improve and keep her beauty have caused her to experiment with all the growing things around her in search of good and lasting beauty products. This pursuit of beauty is as old as the love of beauty.

Few things have been overlooked in the relentless search for maintaining and creating loveliness. The herbs of the field and the very soil itself have been put to use as sources of life so necessary to beauty.

Until recent generations, women had to rely on their own ingenuity in producing cosmetics, for preparation in commercial quantity is a modern innovation. For a time, the novelty and excitement of purchasing creams, lotions and pomades which promised incredible rewards of restored youth turned women away from their homemade cosmetics. But interest has been aroused once again in simple preparations which feed, nourish and soothe the complexion.

A young woman has only to look at her mother's troubled skin and her own and compare them with her grandmother's smooth complexion to realize that grandmother's simple applications must have been better.

Many of the recipes and formulas in this book came from such grandmothers who maintained their exquisite complexions and hair by using homemade concoctions. Other recipes came from younger women in various parts of the world who practice their grandmother's or aunt's or cousin's beauty secrets. These hand-me-down formulas have been added to and improved upon in many instances. Many recipes given were devised in the kitchen by women who felt that if certain foods were good for them taken internally, then quite obviously they would be of benefit used externally. And when used sensibly and with dedication, these various suggestions should go far to ward off the unwelcome aspects of age brought on by neglect and ill-treatment of the body.

There is no reason to suppose that numerical years should unduly decimate one's youthful appearance. With proper care given to all parts of the body, one can remain vitally alive and attractive throughout life. We begin proper care with a nutritionally wise diet that eliminates all non-foods. A non-food is any food that in any way has been processed, refined, preserved chemically or devitalized.

In addition, exercises must be performed in order to keep muscles flexible, ligaments supple, skin tissue elastic and the bloodstream clean. With these attentions given to the body, the discipline of serenity for mental health becomes easier to practice, and life then becomes the joy that reflects itself in beauty.

While these rules are being practiced, one can turn to nature for external applications that will further beautify the body. Only by following this complete program can youth, beauty and health be achieved and maintained.

Age, then, does not have to be the controlling factor in appearance. The disastrous results of poor care for skin and body will soon be evident no matter what the age. Indifference to one's physical condition quickly brings on the debilitation that ages appearance and shortens life.

The women of history who achieved extra years of enjoyment, productive living and satisfaction because they found a formula for extended youth are legendary.

Even when she was approaching fifty, Helen of Troy was able to wield her beauty as though she were a girl of twenty. Juliette Récamier was sixty years old when a thirty-year-old prince attempted suicide because of her resistance to him. Diane de Poitiers commanded as much of her variety of happiness as she desired, so beautiful were her face and figure.

Ninon de Lenclos, everyone's ideal of ageless beauty, was well into her eighties when she enjoyed her last liaison. This scintillating French woman was the envy of women one-third her age, so beautifully did she maintain herself in both mind and body.

In recent times, the late Cecile Sorel, in private life the Comtesse de Ségur, played the role of an eighteen-year-old on the French stage when she was actually sixty-six. Her appearance of youth and freshness was unassailable.

When we speak of youth or a youthful appearance, we are not referring to a *jeune fille* air, or an immaturity of style. Beauty alone is useless unless it reflects the experiences of living. Youth to us means a *joie de vivre*, a natural vitality of body, skin, hair, eyes—and a composed attitude.

Fading and weakness accompany abuse of the body, whereas careful nurturing will prolong the years of beauty and comfort. And even if the body has been mistreated and subjected to the strains and indulgences of today's feverish pace, it is still rarely too late to reverse the ravages of the years. Such a transformation is not only highly possible, but highly probable when the simple laws of nature are used to pave the path to beauty.

So read through this book to get the overall picture of what is possible and helpful in this new field of making your own cosmetics. When you have chosen those formulas you will want to try, buy or collect *all* of the ingredients and have them on hand before beginning your adventure. Save or collect attractive bottles, jars, containers and attractive labels.

When choosing a recipe to prepare, check over the ingredients and eliminate any of those recipes listing items to which you might be allergic—such as egg yolk, orris powder, milk, etc. Learn to adjust the ingredients to meet your own specific requirements. Not every recipe will be for you or bring magical results. This individual selection and adjustment leads to custom-made beauty care for which there is no substitute. Since one of the purposes of making your own cosmetics is to avoid unnecessary and harmful ingredients, you will not have preservatives in these mixtures.

Some will require refrigeration in order to extend their

use. A good rule is to refrigerate any recipe containing edible food, such as eggs, milk, wheat germ, fruit, vegetables, etc. Even so, without chemical preservatives, some of these will keep only a short time. Therefore, prepare them in the smallest quantities possible, and your cosmetics will be as fresh as your food.

Choose a time when you are relaxed and have leisure so that you will enjoy the art of becoming a cosmetic chemist. Fill in empty hours when you are dispirited or alone by making something delightful to improve your appearance and raise your morale. Creating a new self can be fun!

V.C.T.

Contents

Chapter 1	Cleansing and Restoring the Skin	1
Chapter 2	Recipes for Natural Cosmetics	9
Chapter 3	Freckles and Other Spots	25
Chapter 4	Danger: The Sun	33
Chapter 5	Large Pores: Toners and Tighteners	37
Chapter 6	Honey, The Rejuvenator	41
Chapter 7	Herbal Rebuilders	47
Chapter 8	Facial Masques	53
Chapter 9	Lotions and Potions	61
Chapter 10	Hair: How to Grow It, Color It and Keep It	69
Chapter 11	Hand Care and Cures	83
Chapter 12	Bathing for Body and Soul	91
Chapter 13	Beauty Foods	101
Chapter 14	Cleanliness from Within	111
Chapter 15	Exercises for a Perfect Figure	115
Chapter 16	Exercises for Trouble Spots	125
Chapter 17	Eye Care—Exercises and Wrinkle-Chasers	131
Chapter 18	Perfumes, Scents and Potpourris	136
Sources of Ingredients		144
Glossary		146

CHAPTER ONE

Cleansing and Restoring the Skin

An immaculate skin is the first step toward beauty. There is no other beginning. Lack of cleanliness will lead to the common skin disasters over which glamorizing makeup is useless. We don't mean cold-cream clean, but scrub-brush clean, a thorough washing that removes old dead tissues and allows the breath of life to the new and ever-forming cellular growth.

The skin is a long-suffering part of the body. We can abuse it with overdoses of sunshine and allow lashing winds to denude it of moisture until it becomes almost leather-like in appearance and texture. We can coat it with layers of makeup, force it to dispose of body toxins from poor eating habits, and still, properly treated, the skin can be reclaimed again and again.

The results of extreme neglect will eventually have to be recognized. Untreated acne, years of harsh tanning and uncleansed skin grow increasingly difficult to improve. But, almost invariably, the skin responds to simple administrations with renewed health and beauty.

One of the greatest beauty secrets is to know how to clean the skin properly. In our present-day hurry to accomplish all the tasks we impose upon ourselves, we are inclined to give only partial attention to skin cleansing, and too often we rely on creams for the deep-down cleansing that cream can never accomplish.

An invaluable treasure to own, far outweighing the costliest cream, is a complexion brush. Many women shudder at the thought of the supposed violence to delicate skin from washing the face with a brush. But the face eliminates wastes as does the rest of the body. And a gentle rinse, or slathering of cleansing cream, will not remove this debris effectively.

In order to deep-clean the complexion, some method must be used to penetrate filled pores. If properly done, there will be no skin irritation. On the contrary, the stimulation of such a cleansing produces delicate-appearing skin which in fact will be much stronger in resistance than the coarsened scarf skin which harbors bacterial growth and blemishes.

The complexion brush performs this thorough cleansing perfectly. The brush should be of natural bristle, not synthetic. Though the synthetic brush may be hygienic, it is inclined to irritate the skin. Nor can a hairbrush be substituted. The soft, natural-bristle brush is made especially for the face and goes under the name of complexion brush.

Use a pure soap for your facial scrubbing. There are excellent vegetable soaps on the market. Some are protein in composition, of pure nut and vegetable ingredients. All soap used on the body should be of an acid nature. The healthy skin wears an acid mantle at all times that protects it from bacterial infection.

Alkaline soaps and cosmetics rob the skin of this mantle and leave it vulnerable to surface infections and outbreaks. Although soaps are not generally labelled as to whether they are acid or alkaline, there is a simple test you can make to determine if you have the acid soap you require for a properly protected skin.

A strip of Squibb's nitrazine paper applied to a dampened bar of soap or cosmetic will turn a deep blue when it is alkaline in content. On the contrary, an acid preparation will not change the color of the yellow-tinted nitrazine paper, and in this way you will know the qualities of the soap you are testing.

To throw off daily accumulations of waste which are funneled through the skin ducts, keep these channels clean.

Otherwise, clogging from sebaceous matter will produce the blemishes and choked pores that afflict so many skins. Use the complexion brush and non-alkaline soap to produce a competent lather with which to clean every part of the face and neck. Afterward, rinse away every bit of soap and, finally, add a teaspoon of apple cider vinegar to a couple of cups of water in the basin for your last rinse. This restores the natural acid mantle to the skin and acts as a general skin toner.

A papaya mint tea treatment removes skin debris so thoroughly that it seems to leave you with a brand-new skin that pulses with life. If you practice the daily face scrubbing, the papaya mint tea treatment can be used weekly or monthly, according to your needs and the quantity of makeup you use. This tea application can become a part of your beauty schedule with great benefit to the maintenance of your complexion. The tea bags can be purchased through health food mail-order companies or at most health food shops.

To prepare the papaya mint treatment, bring two cups of water to a boil in a clean glass or stainless steel pot or basin. Do not use aluminum. Place two papaya mint teabags in the pot of boiling water. Allow the tea to simmer briefly for a moment or so before removing it from the fire.

Steep the brew for a few minutes. Take a thick white terry cloth toweling face cloth and dip it into the tea. Wring it out just enough to prevent dripping and apply to the face. The liquid should be hot in order to be effective. But it should not burn the skin, and there should be no discomfort. A thick face cloth or one folded double is desirable in order to retain the heat as long as possible. All parts of the face including the forehead, excepting the eye area, should be treated.

The tea solution must be kept warm enough to open pores and help remove the accumulated dead cells from the skin. As the water cools, replace it on the burner and continue the applications for fifteen minutes. The time element is very important and is one of the keys to the success of the treatment. Ten minutes are not enough. A full fifteen minutes are necessary for any benefit.

A word of caution to those with broken red veins. Because of the exceptional fragility of these tiny hair-like veins, hot compresses of any kind are to be avoided. The veins must be strengthened before applying heat or even using a complexion brush.

But for all other complexions, papaya mint tea applications ease off dead skin debris as nothing else will. Of course, oily and average complexions benefit most. Dry skin needs a covering of some nourishing oil after the tea packs.

What is the magic in this simple treatment? For after it is used, the skin actually seems new and feels remarkably smooth. The papaya enzyme absorbs the dead skin tissue which collects in layers on the face. It literally consumes this lifeless covering which smothers the skin beneath and prevents it from shedding dead growth. Unable to breathe, the living skin is held prisoner beneath the hardened scarf skin which no longer has life.

Skin can become porcelain-like in texture after repeated papaya baths. And you can feel it breathe when it is freed of the cluttering debris.

The living organ that is your skin weighs about seven pounds and covers an area of approximately nineteen square feet. This delicate covering is incredibly strong and at the same time a sensitive barometer to the state of your internal health. Though blemished skin can and does develop from external attack or indifference, skin problems often are symptoms of poor nutrition and lack of exercise. More serious ailments stemming from these and other causes also show up in the complexion.

Even dry and oily skin conditions can suggest faulty diet or poor assimilation. An oily skin can be corrected by the elimination of excess animal fats and fried foods from the diet, for instance, while a dry skin responds in the same way to the addition of nuts and vegetable oils. There are also external helps for these problems.

The natural oils taken from nuts, vegetables, seeds and fruits should all be sought by the person with a dry skin. Besides being eaten, they can be applied as topical dressings over a face coated with some moisturizing agent such as water, milk or juice.

Daily use of these nourishing oils can aid in preventing surface drying of the skin and so avoid flaking, peeling and wrinkles. They are highly preferable to commercial cleansers that may have a mineral oil base which can clog the pores and irritate the tissues.

Dry skin can be scrubbed in order to remove the desiccated, flaky top skin debris. But a protective coating should then be applied. Rather than rubbing the oil directly into the dry skin, it is advisable first to use a moisturizer, as we have just suggested. After a thorough cleansing, gently massage milk or cream into the pores. The liquid penetrates and brings much relief.

Allow the cream to settle and dry somewhat before taking a small amount of any nut, fruit or vegetable oil and patting it well into the face and neck. Blot off the excess after five minutes and leave the oil on overnight, or, if more convenient, during the day.

The result of this double application should be a more resilient, youthful skin. If this routine is practiced daily, the softening effects of the milk or cream and oil will go far toward reducing a lined face and smoothing away wrinkles.

For extremely dry skin, melt a teaspoon of sweet butter and beat into it a couple of tablespoons of whole milk. Apply liberally to a clean face and wear as long as your schedule permits. A makeup foundation for dry skin can be achieved by applying a face cloth dipped into water warm enough to open the pores. When the warmth leaves it, dip it into the water again and re-apply. After a couple of minutes of this, dip clean fingers into sesame seed, apricot or other oil and apply to the face, sealing in the bit of moisture needed for plumping up the pores.

A homemade mayonnaise facial is a great help for the parched complexion. If you have time, whip up the mayonnaise yourself and be sure of using only pure foods that are so wonderful for the skin. It is easy enough to make mayonnaise with a blender. The hand method takes longer and is not a guaranteed success, unless you are an old hand at the drop-by-drop beating methods. In case you are not, try a good commercial brand bought at a health food store and beat an egg yolk and a tablespoon of oil into a half cup of it. Set this aside in the refrigerator for a daily application to your face and neck.

Here is a recipe for the homemade variety that ensures the finest ingredients.

MAYONNAISE

1 egg
½ teaspoon sea salt

2 tablespoons lemon juice
or apple cider vinegar
1 cup salad oil

Put one-half cup of the oil and the remaining ingredients into the blender and cover. Blend on the highest speed until thick. Now pour in the remaining oil in a very slow and steady stream while the motor is running. Refrigerate until needed.

Freshly grated corn produces a dry-skin treatment of great value. This easy-to-produce liquid supplies the richness of oil and milk combined. The fresher the ear of corn, the better the results on the skin. Select a young, full-kerneled ear. After husking and removing the silk, run the ear up and down a hand grater. Or you may use a knife instead of a grater. Gather together the kernels and squeeze them through cheesecloth. Pat the resulting corn milk on a freshly cleaned face. Leave it on for a minimum of fifteen minutes and wash off with tepid water without using soap. Blot the skin dry.

Cleansing and Restoring the Skin

An electric juicer will produce the milk from the cut kernels without the need of cheesecloth. If you've squeezed too much, drink the milk not used as a cosmetic. It tastes good and is high in vitamin A and magnesium, both components of good skin care.

The inside of an avocado skin rubbed over a freshly washed face will soften dry skin. The effects of the rich oil will last long after it has been rinsed off with tepid water.

In caring for dry skin it is wise to remove makeup as soon as you can. If early appointments or duties call for makeup, and you can conveniently clean your face afterward, your skin will benefit from a thin application of your night or day cream patted into the skin and all excess taken off. Splash water over the face and blot dry. Sometimes sheer habit causes one to wear makeup all day. At every opportunity allow your skin a chance to breathe or to absorb some nourishing cream or lotion if it is dry.

Oily skin is just as distressing as dry skin. Pores clog easily in excessively oily skin, and any makeup used is inclined to mix with skin oils and make a pudding type of facial covering. Extra face washing and care is of great help in combatting this condition. With daily attention, the disadvantages can be overcome and an easy upkeep routine developed.

After every face scrubbing, use an astringent rinse of apple cider vinegar and water. Mix the solution and keep it handy alongside your wash basin. A half-and-half mixture of the vinegar and water produces excellent results for oily skin. The cleansing acid cuts through residue film and clears the way for healthful complexion breathing. Actually, all types of skin can benefit from the apple cider vinegar rinse, but oily skin especially improves with its use.

After you clean your face thoroughly, try rubbing it with a slice of raw potato. Leave on for several minutes and then remove with a dampened cotton square.

An excellent cleanser for oily skin is the following almond

meal mixture. You can prepare this, keep it beside your wash basin for convenience and dip into it every evening for deep-down skin cleansing.

ALMOND-MEAL CLEANSER

½ cup almond meal
½ cup Indian cornmeal
½ cup grated castile or vegetable protein soap

Mix together thoroughly without adding a liquid. When you are ready to clean your face, dip into the jar for a tiny palmful. Add enough water to combine the dry ingredients and carefully rub into the skin. Be careful not to irritate sensitive tissue, but do create enough friction to cleanse and stimulate.

Rinse off with tepid water and blot dry. Use an apple cider vinegar rinse and dry again.

A simplified method is to use edible almond butter available in jars in health food stores. It is an excellent pore cleanser.

CHAPTER TWO

Recipes for Natural Cosmetics

Many women are surprised to learn that it is possible to become one's own beautician and produce a fine complexion without ever buying a pot of cream or bottle of lotion. Since we are so accustomed to searching for a wonder cream that will conceal, remove or destroy skin defects, habit dies hard. It is still considered far easier to study a cosmetic counter, sniff the contents of a cream jar and accept its stated claims.

But how often have the promised results materialized? So one drifts on to another brand of pretty, sweet-smelling potion and awaits results before pushing that jar, too, to the back of the shelf.

Smooth, delicate and even exquisite complexions can be uncovered from beneath unattractive skin surfaces by turning to simple preparations you can mix in your own kitchen. In fact, many of the ingredients can be found in your kitchen. Others will have to be sought out. But the results of an improved skin make the effort more than worthwhile. It is an absolute joy to make natural, unchemicalized beauty preparations and be rewarded by a complexion that appears years younger than it really is or has appeared to be in many years.

Removal of the tired, lifeless complexion requires discipline and good living habits, besides the use of cosmetics based on natural ingredients. There is no discomfort attached to the process. Actually, both beauty and health increase when one follows the natural pathway instead of settling for the artificially contrived beauty that washes off with soap and water.

Remember, the following recipes lack the usual preservatives or chemical additives. A homemade, natural skin food should not be expected to be less perishable than the food you eat. So make up small quantities of complexion creams, lotions and milks. Refrigerate when necessary and use daily for good results.

Ingredients such as cocoa butter, rose water and lanolin can be found in most pharmacies. The lanolin itself should be the hydrous type, which is already mixed with water. Anhydrous lanolin requires the addition of a suitable amount of liquid.

Almond oil, sesame, apricot and any other nut, vegetable or fruit oil can be purchased through health food shops and mail-order health companies.

Raw, green, cold-pressed olive oil has not been heated or cooked for preservative reasons. Our purpose in specifying the unprocessed oils is to insure having the ingredients at their nutritive best for the finest results. However, you may substitute virgin olive oil for the cold-pressed oil if you cannot find the other.

Benzoin, gum arabic, frankincense and orris root should be obtainable through a pharmacy. If not, you will have to locate one of the older herbal houses that specializes in these products and usually supplies them through a mail order. Indiana Botanic Gardens in Hammond, Indiana, is one such place.

For some ingredients in the following recipes, such as orange water, a gourmet shop is usually a help. Rose water is also obtainable in some of these shops. (They sell it for cooking purposes, but as long as it is pure rose water, it is usable as a cosmetic also.)

Ethyl alcohol is specified for use in the recipes in this book to distinguish it from isopropyl alcohol. While both are rubbing alcohols, ethyl alcohol is more suitable because of its less pungent odor.

While the botanic gardens carry rose geranium oils, rose

water and other scenting mediums including elder flower blossoms, you can sometimes obtain these from a pharmacy.

Try looking around your own home for many of your ingredients. There are dandelions on the lawn and roses in the garden (unsprayed we hope; sprayed roses just won't do). Check the trees in your neighborhood. Sometimes you can find an elder tree that will supply you with the scented blossoms to be used fresh and to dry for later on.

In the recipes for aromatic vinegar, while we prefer apple cider vinegar to the more refined white vinegar, the scent is stronger and more difficult to conceal. Whichever vinegar you use, be sure to store the aromatics in glass containers.

Many of the old recipes given me specified the use of rainwater. But because of the dangers of fallout liberally lacing such water nowadays, and the numerous other disadvantages of trying to collect one's own soft rainwater, we have substituted either mineral or purified water.

When using nut meats, such as almonds, buy the ones in the shell and shell them yourself. The oils in the opened varieties begin oxidizing upon exposure to the air, and as a consequence, the nut meats are inclined to be rancid. It takes a bit longer to shell them yourself, but your creams will be all the better for it.

Now we are ready for these fascinating formulas. Experiment with them. Keep notes and repeat recipes you find best for your skin and needs.

NINA'S NIGHT CREAM

2 tablespoons cocoa butter
3 tablespoons almond oil
2 tablespoons lanolin

2 teaspoons rose water
½ teaspoon honey

Place the first three ingredients in a glass custard dish in a pan of hot water over a low flame. Stir the contents with a wooden spoon until they are melted and smooth. Remove the custard cup from the pan and add two teaspoons of rose water and one-half teaspoon honey. Cool the mixture and then beat until well blended.

Pour the resulting cream into a small container.

Apply Nina's night cream nightly, or daily, for the best results. Use for stubborn wrinkles and lines on both face and throat.

COCOA BUTTER CREAM FOR THE THROAT

2 tablespoons cocoa butter
2 tablespoons lanolin
4 tablespoons safflower oil

Measure all ingredients into a non-metallic pot and heat over boiling water to a liquid state. Stir thoroughly to blend and pour into small jar to keep.

An excellent cream for dry, crepey throat areas. Best results come from washing the throat area and allowing it to remain a bit moist. Then quickly apply a thin covering of the cream in order to capture the moisture.

STRAWBERRY MAINTENANCE CREAM

½ cup freshly squeezed strawberry juice
1 soupspoon lanolin
1 soupspoon oatmeal flour

To obtain the strawberry juice, use less than one cup of freshly picked strawberries. Wash carefully and shake off excess water. Crush berries through a cheesecloth into a cup. Heat the lanolin in a glass custard cup placed in a pan of hot water over a low flame. To the melted lanolin, add the oatmeal flour. Stir until dissolved and well blended. Mix in the strawberry juice and beat until creamy before removing from the heat. Cool and store in a clean jar with a lid. Refrigerate when not in use.

APRICOT CLEANSING CREAM

4 tablespoons apricot oil
2 tablespoons sweet butter
2 tablespoons sesame seed oil
1 tablespoon purified water

Beat the ingredients with an egg beater until completely blended. Pour into a lidded jar and use nightly as a cleansing cream. Apricot cleansing cream also softens and maintains the skin.

LETTUCE COMPLEXION CREAM

1 cup young lettuce
½ cup lanolin

2 drops rose geranium oil or perfume

Wash the lettuce and cut into fine strips. Heat the lanolin in a non-metallic container over boiling water until it is liquid. Add the lettuce and continue to heat a few minutes longer. Remove from heat and add scent. Beat until cold and pack into small jars.

Lettuce is useful in refining the skin in addition to its nourishing and soothing qualities.

GYPSY ELDER FLOWER CREAM

1 tablespoon lanolin
6 ounces sweet almond oil

1 cup elder flowers

Pick fresh elder flowers in full, sweet bloom or purchase from the herbal tea department in a health food store. Melt the lanolin in a glass bowl set into a pan of hot water. Mix in the sweet almond oil and blend well. Add the elder flower petals and simmer for twenty to thirty minutes. Cool and strain in order to remove the petals. Pack in a clean jar with a lid.

Wandering gypsies had access to the sweetly scented elder flowers for this cream. With its help they maintained their blemish-free complexions which could withstand the rigors of many climates. One of the elder flower's many virtues, if used daily, is its ability to help smooth a lined face. Tea, made from the blossoms, is considered a calming brew for the nerves.

SESAME OIL CLEANSING CREAM

2 tablespoons sesame seed oil
4 tablespoons raw green pressed olive oil

2 tablespoons vegetable shortening, without preservatives
2 drops scented oil

Beat ingredients together until well blended, and place in a lidded jar. Rub gently into the face and neck and remove with cotton squares.

ELDER FLOWER CLEANSING CREAM

1 teaspoon grated vegetable soap
2 tablespoons cocoa butter
1 teaspoon corn oil
4 tablespoons sesame seed oil
2 tablespoons elder flower water

Melt grated soap in custard cup over hot water. Add cocoa butter, oils and elder flower water. Beat together until thoroughly blended and store in a lidded jar.

APRICOT WRINKLE-ERASER CREAM

2 tablespoons lanolin
1 tablespoon apricot oil
1 teaspoon lemon juice
3 drops simple tincture benzoin

Melt lanolin in custard cup in pan of water over low heat. Beat in apricot oil and lemon juice until well blended. Add benzoin and beat again.

WRINKLE CREAM I

1 teaspoon powdered sweet almond
¼ teaspoon powdered cloves
¼ teaspoon powdered nutmeg
½ ounce rose water

Mix almond, cloves and nutmeg thoroughly and allow to stand forty-eight hours, shaking now and then to mix. Add one-half ounce rose water. Strain the mixture through a coarse cloth. Apply at night and rinse off in the morning with warm water. Apply sweet almond oil and rub in gently afterwards.

FOREHEAD WRINKLES

Mix equal parts of alcohol and egg white and apply to the forehead. Allow to dry on. Rinse away with warm water.

SKIN SOFTENER

3 tablespoons sweet almond oil
2 tablespoons lanolin

Few drops simple tincture of benzoin

Put all three ingredients into a bottle and shake vigorously until well blended.

ANTI-WRINKLE CREAM

¼ teaspoon pulverized gum benzoin

¼ teaspoon gum arabic
¼ teaspoon frankincense

Dissolve the above in one pint of alcohol. Add:

1 teaspoon pulverized pine nut kernels
1 teaspoon pulverized sweet almonds

¼ teaspoon pulverized cloves
¼ teaspoon pulverized nutmeg

Allow the mixture to steep for two days, stirring it twice each day before adding ¼ cup rose water. Distill to half the quantity.

If you do not have a distilling apparatus, fasten a rubber tube to the spout of a tea kettle containing the mixture. Lay the tube in a pan of ice cubes and put the other end in a glass jar where the moisture will collect. If you are one of the many who now owns a small water distiller, by all means take advantage of it.

Many of the old recipes required a complete distilling apparatus in the home. If you do not have such an apparatus, the above homemade substitute can be quite effective and opens up an enormous field of possibilities to the enthusiast of homemade distillations.

REFINING PASTE

3 ounces ground barley
1 ounce honey

1 egg white, unbeaten

Mix all three ingredients until a well-blended and smooth paste is formed. Store in a covered jar and use nightly. Spread on the cheeks, nose, forehead and chin and gently rub into the skin. Rinse off in the morning with warm water. Oil or cream-feed the skin afterward.

ALMOND PASTE

4 ounces blanched almonds   rose water
1 egg white

Rub the almonds to a smooth paste. Add the unbeaten egg white and enough rose water to make a paste of a spreadable consistency. Use as a refining and nourishing skin paste.

ALMOND PASTE #2

4 ounces powdered almonds   3 ounces lemon juice
3 ounces sweet almond oil   rose water

Beat the almond oil into the powdered almonds. Add the lemon juice and continue to blend. Add enough rose water to bring to a spreadable consistency. Use as a complexion paste for cleansing that also refines and tones.

WRINKLE ERADICATOR

Dip strips of gauze into the unbeaten white of an egg. Apply in the opposite direction of lines on the face. Smooth out the gauze and hold it in place until the cloth dries. Use once daily until lines lessen. Dampen thoroughly with warm water before removing.

BARLEY FLOUR FOR IMPROVING THE COMPLEXION

1 ounce barley flour   honey
1 ounce blanched almonds

Pulverize the almonds and mix with the barley flour. Add enough honey to make a smooth paste. Apply and leave on a minimum of thirty minutes. Remove with warm water.

Recipes for Natural Cosmetics

KEEPING CREAM

2 tablespoons lanolin
1 tablespoon olive oil
1 tablespoon corn oil
1 tablespoon purified water
Few drops of scent if desired

Melt the lanolin in a custard cup in a pan of hot water over a low flame. Add the oils slowly, beating all the while with a wooden spoon. Continue to beat until the mixture emulsifies. Add perfume. Store in a covered jar, use nightly for two weeks and then notice the velvety texture of your skin. This recipe is from a friend working abroad for the U.S. Government. She devised the cream after living and working in hot and cold countries. She found that it kept wrinkles under control in both climates.

SKIN FOOD CREAM

3 tablespoons wheat germ oil
1 teaspoon apple cider vinegar
3 tablespoons sesame seed oil

Beat together until well blended. Apply nightly after thoroughly scrubbing the face, followed by a face cloth steaming for a minute or two. Leave the cream on all night and remove the following morning by bathing in warm water and using an apple cider vinegar rinse.

NECK CREAM

1 tablespoon wheat germ oil
1 teaspoon malt extract
1 teaspoon honey

Beat all ingredients together until well blended. Apply nightly to a thoroughly cleansed throat and neck, using upward sweeping motions. The vitamin E in the wheat germ oil stimulates the tissue and helps to remove sagging neck folds. Use nightly for several months for best results.

ALMOND MEAL FOR PORE CLEANSING

Skin a pound of almonds by plunging them into hot water and then cold. A large strainer is ideal for this, for it enables you to lower the basket part into the two waters. Mash the blanched almonds in a mortar. You can use a special nut grinder or try the fastest speed on a blender. A good substitute for a mortar and pestle is a strong earthenware or wooden bowl, and an old china doorknob to use as the pestle, or grinder. When you have a very fine paste, mix this with enough rose water to form a milky consistency. Strain this through gauze.

Return the mixture remaining in the cloth to the mortar and mash in the same manner. Add the strained liquid, mix and strain once more. Repeat until the whole mixture will sift through gauze.

Place the almond mixture in the top part of a double boiler and allow to remain over the heat until all the moisture has evaporated. Spread out on a clean cloth and when the mixture is completely dry to the touch, store in a clean jar and use as needed for deep pore cleansing.

VARIETY SKIN FOOD CREAMS

LEMON CREAM

1 tablespoon softened sweet butter

1 tablespoon fresh lemon juice

STRAWBERRY CREAM

1 tablespoon softened sweet butter

1 tablespoon strawberry pulp

CORN CREAM

1 tablespoon softened sweet butter

1 tablespoon milk from freshly grated corn

CUCUMBER CREAM

1 tablespoon softened sweet butter

1 tablespoon cucumber juice

EGG CREAM

1 tablespoon softened sweet butter

1 teaspoon egg yolk

To make these creams, beat the butter and fruit, vegetable pulp, juice or egg yolk together with a fork until the juice and butter are well emulsified. Apply to a clean face and neck and allow to remain for a minimum of fifteen minutes. Many kinds of food can be used in this recipe. Use fresh foods that are nourishing and spreadable. Rinse off with warm water and splash an astringent on the face before blotting off.

Butter in these recipes offers a good source of vitamin A for distressed skin, while the various fruits and vegetables add their nourishing qualitities.

COMPLEXION WASH

½ teaspoon powdered benzoin
½ teaspoon nutmeg oil

6 drops orange blossom tea
1 pint sherry

Shake all the ingredients together and bottle. Use every morning and every night for a clear complexion.

This is an old Spanish recipe used by women who cherished a good complexion. As you try various recipes you may find that some of the ingredients will work better if they are decreased in quantity. If this is the case, then adjust the recipe to suit your own personal needs.

ALMOND COMPLEXION WASH

3 tablespoons sweet almond oil

3 tablespoons rose water
juice of two lemons

Beat the ingredients together until well blended. Apply at night and allow to dry on the skin without blotting. Wash off in the morning with warm water.

Almond oil is one of the finest complexion oils, and its softening qualities have been noted for centuries. This easy-to-use complexion wash also softens and reduces pores.

ELDER FLOWER RINSE

1 cup elder flowers, fresh or dried
1 pint boiling water

Place the elder flowers in a bowl. Pour the boiling water over the blossoms and leave to steep overnight. Strain into a bottle and cap.

For a lemon and elder flower rinse, add the juice of one lemon to the strained elder flower water and shake vigorously. Use as a toning lotion after cleansing the skin, the same as the plain elder flower rinse.

ROSE WATER

2 cups sweetest rose petals
1 pint purified water
¼ pound sugar

Put all ingredients into an earthenware pot and allow to steep together for an hour. Have another earthenware pot waiting, and pour the solution from the first pot into the second one. Continue this process until the water takes on the scent of roses. Strain and keep in a cool place.

This was one of the methods used to make rose water in the seventeenth century. While the pouring requires some effort, the results are good. Another way to make rose water is to pick three cups of heavily scented rose petals just after the sun has dried the morning dew. Pour three cups of boiling water over them and allow the concoction to steep in a glass or porcelain container for two days, stirring frequently. Strain and bottle for use.

Rose water has a very delicate, slight fragrance. Do not confuse it with the more concentrated rose oils and rose perfumes.

BARLEY ASTRINGENT

2 tablespoons non-pearled barley
½ pint water
5 drops Balsam of Tolu

Boil the barley and water together until a soft mixture is formed. Strain and add the balsam. Shake well. Use as a tonic for oily skin.

TONIC FOR ENLARGED PORES

Use equal parts of alcohol and witch hazel, shaken together vigorously to mix. Apply with a soft cloth and allow to dry on the skin.

ORANGE FLOWER WATER FOR PIMPLES

3 ounces orange flower water
¼ teaspoon simple tincture of benzoin

Mix the benzoin drop by drop into the orange flower water. Shake well until completely blended and milky. Pour a small amount onto a cotton square and gently pat onto the face. If there is a drawing sensation to the skin, add more orange flower water. There should be no discomfort felt in using this solution. A pulling sensation indicates that the solution is too strong.

This lotion can be used to advantage for superficial eruptions because of its drying qualities.

AROMATIC VINEGARS FOR TONING THE SKIN

2 pints washed and hulled strawberries
1 pint vinegar

Place the strawberries in a glass or porcelain container with the vinegar and cover. Allow to steep for one week, then strain into bottles and cap. Do not use metal in preparing or storing vinegar rinses.

RASPBERRY VINEGAR

2 cups raspberries
1 cup scented rose petals
1 teaspoon honey

Immerse the above in one quart vinegar and steep for one month. Filter and use diluted half and half with water as a skin toner.

ROSE VINEGAR

4 cups dried red rose leaves   ½ cup essence of rose
1 pint vinegar

Mix the ingredients together in a glass jar and cover with a lid. Allow to stand two or three weeks, during which time shake the jar frequently. Filter and place in a glass bottle or jar with a cap or lid.

    To make essence of rose: A quick method for producing this strong scent requires bringing to a boil the amount of distilled water required—in this case one-half cup—and stirring in briskly a few drops of rose compound oil. Cool and add to the recipe.

MILK VINEGAR

4 tablespoons alcohol   3 tablespoons vinegar
3 tablespoons tincture of
   benzoin

Mix together and let stand for a week. Slowly pour through filtering paper and bottle. Dilute with water when ready to use.

PEPPERMINT VINEGAR FOR SKIN TIGHTENING

1 pint vinegar   1 cup mint leaves
1 pint purified water

Place all ingredients in a glass or enamel cooking pot and bring to a boil before removing from the heat. Pour into a glass jar and allow to steep uncovered for four days. Strain and bottle.

LAVENDER VINEGAR WATER

2 handfuls of lavender   1 pint vinegar
   flowers   1 ounce powdered orris root

Steep together for three weeks and strain. Bottle for use.

    Aromatic vinegar rinses afford a pleasant way to tone the skin with a scented water that is beneficial in its acid content. All vinegar rinses must be diluted before using. Usually a half-and-half dilution, that is, half rinse and half water, makes a very satisfactory combination. If this proves too strong, simply add more water.

CARROT AND BEET ROOT POWDER

Slice and scrape six raw carrots and half a beet. Squeeze through a muslin bag. Mix the resulting juice with three ounces of cornstarch. Spread onto a flat enamel dish and place in the sun, stirring occasionally, until all the moisture is evaporated. This produces a prettily tinted powder.

EGGSHELL POWDER

Save until you have a small basketful of egg shells. Wash them thoroughly and remove all traces of the albumen. Crush the shells to a powder either in a mortar with a pestle or with a rolling pin on a flat surface. Sift the powder and recrush until it is of the finest consistency. Mix the finely powdered shell with a little cologne water and allow to dry. When the powder is entirely dry, sift again. This should result in a soft, creamy powder.

OLIVE OIL FACIAL BATH FOR DRY SKIN

You must lie down for this. First scrub the face and rinse off all soap. Splash with a vinegar water rinse and blot dry. Have waiting three tablespoons of warm olive oil, enough opened cotton squares to cover the face, and a small towel that has been soaked in hot water and wrung out. Dip cotton squares into the oil and squeeze out excess. Lie down and place the squares carefully over the entire face. Then place the hot towel over the pieces of cotton, to cover all the face except the nostrils. The heat of the moist towel will help the oil to penetrate. After the towel cools, remove it and the oiled cotton squares. Towel off the excess oil and complete the facial with a mild vinegar rinse. Blot dry.

CHAPTER THREE

Freckles and Other Spots

In the days when a beautiful skin had to be as creamy as a bowl of sifted rice flour, freckles put one in the position of a lost Cinderella. Not any more. Beauty is more readily recognized now in its maintenance and charm than by any preconceived notions of hue or quality.

A smattering of freckles can become an asset, just as one can emphasize beauty around too-wide-set eyes, an elongated face or anything else that varies from the popular concept of perfection. At the same time, some of those who are heavily endowed with freckles might prefer a less lavish display and want to tone them down.

Women have battled freckles for centuries and come up with some interesting and fairly effective methods of dealing with them. With persistent treatment, they can often be lightened. But this is really about as much as one can hope for.

Freckles can usually be divided into two classes: summer freckles, which are brought out on fair-skinned persons during exposure to the more intense rays of the sun and which gradually disappear when the season is over, and winter freckles which are permanent. Even these can be faded somewhat, with daily attention given to bleaching and reducing their intensity.

There are many commercial products on the market to fade freckles. But most of them, if not all, depend for their effect on a peeling of the skin surface containing the unwanted pigment. It would seem safer by far to try a simple, organic approach and end up not only with a lightened pigmentation, but also a skin that is not irritated or otherwise damaged.

After using any of the bleaches for freckles or skin discoloration recommended here, apply cream or oil in order to avoid irritation to sensitive tissues. Then if any irritation results, you should discontinue the applications and return to the practice later with a weaker mixture or adjusted combinations.

Daily scrubbing with a complexion brush is considered a good treatment for freckles, since scrubbing increases the circulation of the blood. An early beauty researcher, Harriet Hubbard Ayer, says she found this to be one of the best methods of eliminating heavy deposits of freckles.

Don't actually try to scrub away the spots themselves, however. Increased circulation helps, but the skin could also be damaged by an over-enthusiastic approach.

METHODS TO REMOVE FRECKLES

Vitamin C masques have been noted for effectively removing light freckles and toning down darker ones. In any application to the face or body, a natural, rather than synthetic, vitamin source should be used. Such sources of vitamin C are available from acerola berries or unsweetened rose hip powder.

The powder is easier to work with, but, in the absence of that, crush enough tablets to make a small amount of paste when combined with cucumber juice. Apply this paste to a well-scrubbed and rinsed face and allow it to remain on for ten or fifteen minutes. Repeat daily.

Simple foods used externally as bleaches avoid the possible injurious effects of the chemicals in commercial freckle-remover creams. The following mixture is safe and rewarding:

¼ cup of buttermilk or sour milk	½ teaspoon of freshly grated horseradish
	1 tablespoon of cornmeal

Mix the three ingredients together thoroughly into a loose paste and spread between two layers of thin muslin or cheesecloth. Taking care to avoid the areas around the eyes, place the cloth over the freckles and allow it to remain on as long as there is no irritation produced, but for no more than an hour. Repeat daily, or every other day, until the freckles fade.

More sensitive skins respond to the following recipe where the horseradish's strength is absorbed into the milk, yet the horseradish itself never touches the skin. Scrape the horseradish into a cup of sour milk and allow it to stand at room temperature for twelve hours. Strain and apply two or three times a day until the freckles fade somewhat.

Lighter freckles can be controlled to some degree by frequent use of diluted lemon juice left on overnight and rinsed away in the morning. The proportion of pure lemon juice to purified water must be adjusted according to the skin's sensitivity. A drop or two of pure honey can also be added to the lotion. Be very sure to cream the skin after removal of this acid type of application.

There are other simple home preparations which, being based on animal or vegetable acid, should not be harmful. But of course, since every skin varies in its needs, any bleach designed to remove discoloration or freckles must be used with some amount of caution.

With that in mind, the following recipe of Madame de Maintenon, the celebrated mistress of Louis XIV of France, is enticing. It seems that she had one flaw in her incredibly beautiful appearance. At least, freckles were considered flaws in her day and she worked just as hard with this recipe as Marie Antoinette later worked with buttermilk for removing suntan.

MADAME DE MAINTENON'S FRECKLE CREAM

1 ounce grated Venice soap (use a good castile soap)
3 tablespoons distilled water
3 teaspoons lemon juice
¼ ounce oil of bitter almonds
¼ teaspoon cream of tartar
3 drops olive oil

Grate the soap into the water and melt in the top of a double boiler over low heat. Simmer until the water has evaporated and only the soap remains. Remove the boiler from the heat and stir in the lemon juice, cream of tartar, oil of bitter almonds and the olive oil.

This mixture was applied at night and rinsed away in the morning. But it might be wise to try a tiny bit during the day, checking frequently for any allergic reactions. Madame de Maintenon apparently held onto her beauty and her king an impressive number of years, but her freckle night cream might not work for everyone. Try a patch test on one or two freckles before branching out to complete coverage.

Another recipe that softens the skin as it removes freckles is a tolu and benzoin combination. These resinous liquids are a bit sticky to work with, but they have pleasing qualities, and benzoin can even be considered an antiseptic lotion in its effective use on the complexion. Both tolu and benzoin whiten the skin.

¼ cup tincture of tolu*   1½ teaspoons oil of rosemary
½ cup tincture of benzoin   Distilled water

Mix all ingredients together thoroughly by placing in a jar and shaking well. When ready to use, put one teaspoon of this mixture in 3 ounces of distilled water and apply to the face with a soft sponge two or three times a day.

Tincture of tolu (for use in above recipe)
  Steep ½ ounce balsam of Tolu with 4 ounces of brandy for several days. Shake occasionally during this time, then strain and bottle.

A successful freckle remedy completely lacking in a pleasant scent is a mixture of apple cider vinegar and milk. Shake together in a bottle one cup of vinegar, one cup of distilled water and one cup of milk. Shake vigorously each evening and apply to the face before retiring. Allow it to dry on the skin, without blotting. Remove each morning with tepid water and use a brisk movement with a towel to dry.

Almond meal and its oil, which serve so very many cosmetic purposes, have long been used to fade freckles. Soften the skin with almond paste (it can be bought as almond butter for a food in health stores), rinse and then apply lemon juice, leaving this on until it dries. Rinse again and apply a rich cream.

AIDS FOR OTHER SKIN DISCOLORATIONS

Other discolorations of the skin can stem from systemic causes, drugs, overexposure to the sun's rays, external applications of chemicals from synthetic perfumes or other cosmetics. Even frequent use of birth control pills has been known to tinge the complexion with brown pigmented areas.

In earlier times, and also in some modern day preparations, flowers of sulphur has been considered helpful in toning down the depth of some skin discolorations. However, though pharmacists say it can be used safely in a mild solution of lemon juice and water, the odor is far too objectionable.

Cranberry juice is a gentle but effective bleach for discolored skins. You can either prepare your own, which is preferable, or buy the bottled, unsweetened cranberry juice in a health food store and use it daily. In fact, two or more applications daily would be a good schedule to follow. Allow the juice to dry on the skin before rinsing it away.

Other fruits can be used in the same manner. Lemon juice will work in the same way as with freckles. Dried apricots, stewed in water without adding any sweetening, is another effective bleach.

Cook the apricots until completely soft, after soaking them overnight, and mash to a pulpy consistency. Apply to the face and neck while lying down. Allow the mash to work at bleaching for twenty-five to thirty minutes before removing it and rinsing the face and neck.

Plain buttermilk, rather than the stronger combination with horseradish used for freckles, is a fine bleach. Get raw certified buttermilk if you possibly can, but the modern kind will also do. Be lavish with the buttermilk when applying it, and with a padded gauze or cotton swab, layer both face and neck. Set aside an hour for this and dab on the buttermilk from time to time.

This is not a comfortable treatment, but its bleaching and unifying of skin tones make it worth the momentary soggy discomfort. Marie Antoinette found this method of removing discoloration from her skin so effective that she daily lathered her face, neck, bosom, shoulders and arms with compresses of buttermilk. This was to counteract her hours spent in the sun around her *hammeau*, or little farm.

It was here she played at being a milkmaid during the summer months. Evenings found her coiffed and gowned with gleaming skin bared to a low decolletage. She was able to lead this double life because of her daily buttermilk sponges which removed the effects of the sun's rays from her delicate skin.

Yogurt also attacks uneven color distribution and helps produce a finer skin texture at the same time. Pat on a thick covering of yogurt and allow it to remain for twenty-five to thirty minutes, or until it dries. Rinse away and soothe the skin with a rose water, elder flower or orange water rinse. If you prefer, you can leave the yogurt on overnight for even better results and wash it away in the morning.

A Spanish recipe for combatting the results of the Castilian sun on fine Spanish complexions calls for one egg white and its measure equivalent of lemon juice beaten together and heated over hot water, stirring as it thickens. This is cooled and applied to a clean face and left on for an hour or more for best results.

Cucumber and parsley juice mixed together and applied several times a day will also lighten the skin considerably without the caustic action of stronger bleaches. While the organic method is slower, it is not only safer, but also brings dividends of toning, strengthening and nourishing the skin.

For bleaching purposes, use parsley juice instead of cucumber as you would for freckles, with natural vitamin C powder made into a thin paste.

Paint this on the discolored areas and allow to remain until dry before rinsing off. The thin paste can be used two or three times a week. Because of the potency of the vitamin C powder, the skin should always be carefully rinsed afterward, and the film of oil or cream never forgotten.

In medieval days, fairness of complexion was just as much sought as today. Women then were more inclined to know and trust nature as a remedial source. They soaked tansy leaves in buttermilk for the space of a week, and the resulting liquid was strained and used as a wash for their complexions. One comes across the tansy plant growing in specialized herb gardens, but, unfortunately, it seems to have become rare. However, if you do find tansy, the lotion is effective.

Slightly modified, the apple cider vinegar, water and milk mixture used on freckles is also good to achieve an overall even coloring to the skin. Simply use three-fourths of a cup of vinegar, instead of a cup, and apply as for freckles.

CHAPTER FOUR

Danger: The Sun

For generations now, summer beauty has meant suntanned beauty. The deeper the bronze, the greater the appreciation. But recent discoveries have revealed the dangers from the long hours of exposure required to develop a deep tan.

Anyone who strives for a good complexion and resilient skin would do well to avoid overexposure to sunlight. Sun worshippers lead the list in premature aging as well as skin cancer. While a moderate amount of sunshine is beneficial and even necessary for good health and radiant beauty, that amount should be carefully supervised and never permitted to become an overdose.

Sunlight is now known to be more responsible for aging of the skin than the numerical years themselves. All of the manifestations of age come to the overexposed complexion. With great quantities of sunlight, the skin begins to dry. As the oils and moisture disappear, wrinkles form. Bit by bit, all vestiges of youth will leave the skin that is overexposed to the sun's rays without concern for the damaging effects.

Sun-damaged skin does not spring back with elasticity as a more protected skin will. When there is a tendency toward freckling, the skin is even more susceptible to overexposure. Brown spots, so detested by women everywhere, also plague the skin that is not shielded from the sun's ultraviolet radiation.

No beauty can survive dry, withered, leather-like skin. Once the covering of the body has been severely damaged, one cannot expect to remove all of the harm done by the dry burn of the sun, though eventually one may coax back a less withered skin. Sometimes the destruction may not show itself for some years. But skin cancer can eventually appear, and even one case of bad sunburn can create susceptibility to this disease.

Tanning in itself is brought about by an increase in the pigment, melanin, which responds to the sun's heat on the skin. This creates the color considered so fashionable by so many. After overdoses of the sun, the blood vessels become enlarged, followed by painful, red sunburn.

A complexion that has been protected from the sun's rays presents a more youthful appearance than the over-baked skin. And the years of maintaining fresh, young skin will be longer for those who have guarded it well. Even the young can suffer ill effects from overdoses of the sun. The fact that the skin bounces back in youth gives one a sense of overconfidence. And by the time its owner realizes that her skin has lost its restorative power, she is already in trouble.

The fact that women who are seriously interested in their appearance court the sun so avidly and with such determination seems foolish in itself. What possible value can there be in coating and cooking the skin until it changes color and texture? For surely the soft, lustrous skin that is so pleasant to touch cannot be expected to endure such abuse. The skin becomes thicker and loses much of its vitality even as it tans.

Overexposed skin is damaged skin, and repeated exposure reduces the skin's ability to heal.

Women who retain their beauty the longest are usually the ones who suffer the most from extended sun exposure and, consequently, avoid it. Redheads and the extremely fair-skinned are usually so sensitive to the sun's rays that they have to devise protective habits and shields against exposure.

These women at fifty and sixty have the appearance of much younger women. But the woman who has abused her skin with indiscriminate sunbathing has a youthful appearance only in the areas of her body that are shielded completely from the sun's rays: her buttocks, and now, in the day of the bikini, the lower part of her abdomen only. This should be proof enough!

Another proof that excess sun toughens and spoils a fine complexion is that women in rainier, less sunshiny areas retain their skin beauty far longer than those living in tropical or semi-tropical areas. The women of England, Scotland, Ireland and the islands off their coasts have delicate skin tones that remain moist and supple long after their counterparts in torrid zone areas have developed seared skin riddled with senescent mottling.

A moderate amount of sun is desirable, as we know. When we speak of avoiding the sun, we do not mean that one must be pallid in order to avoid aging symptoms. But normal rather than planned exposure should be the aim. This eliminates long hours spent lying on a beach or at a pool absorbing the sun's full rays. It also means wearing a brimmed hat if regular time is spent in gardening.

In spite of knowing the effects of exposure to the sun, there are those who are indifferent to the results, or to whom a "beautiful tan" is more important than their health. To them, we offer the following recipes to lessen the damaging effects.

Beat the yolk of an egg until it is lemon colored. Beat in very slowly one cup of olive oil or sesame seed oil and continue beating until the liquid becomes thickened. Add one tablespoon of apple cider vinegar and one tablespoon of wheat germ oil and blend together. Apply to all parts of the body to be exposed to the sun.

The oils and vinegar solution of this recipe helps in getting a safer tan and hastens the tanning process.

Cocoa butter, available from drugstores for pennies, rubbed on the skin before an overall exposure to the sun is excellent, even though you smell a bit chocolaty.

Just a mixture of salad oil and apple cider vinegar provides a slightly protective shield against the sun. And for those who find themselves stinging from too much sun, equal parts of baking soda and water patted onto the sunburned areas and left on for half an hour is supposed to bring relief. Rinse away with tepid water.

Or beat the white of an egg with one teaspoon of castor oil and smooth it over burned skin as a healing lotion.

CHAPTER FIVE

Large Pores: Toners and Tighteners

An otherwise attractive appearance can be nullified by noticeable, crater-like pore openings. Refining pores cannot be accomplished in a hurry. It is advisable to go slowly, be patient and be absolutely unfailing in daily administrations. In time, with the proper care, the pores should be greatly reduced and a more attractive complexion produced. In addition to a lovelier appearance, reducing the size of the pores also lessens the possibility of skin infection. Experiment with abrasive recipes very cautiously and avoid them if your skin is unduly sensitive.

One approach toward this problem is very simple: use iced salt water twice a day. Rub the solution gently across the enlarged pore area without irritating the skin. Rinse away and pat dry. Apply a soothing oil to the area, and blot away any excess.

A granular abrasive is usually helpful in reducing oversize pores, and cornmeal serves well here. Indian cornmeal is far better to work with than the standard meal as it is milled finer and is not so coarse.

Mix equal quantities of cornmeal and finely grated castile soap together and keep in a covered container by the wash basin. Use twice daily unless skin sensitivity dictates otherwise. Take enough of the mixture in your palm to produce a paste when mixed with a little water. Dip your washcloth into the paste and gently rub in upward motions across the pore areas. Rinse well and blot dry.

With any of these treatments, it is helpful to use a final

rinse of equal quantities of apple cider vinegar and cool water to tighten the pores.

Sea salt is another helpful measure in reducing pore openings, if used cautiously. In time, a smooth, almost marble-like skin texture can be produced if the sea salt is applied faithfully. Use the fine grade of sea salt coming from the Pacific rather than the coarser quality that would prove damaging to facial tissues. Wet the face and the salt and gently rub upward in and around the face and neck area just briefly. Rinse away with warm, then cool water, and blot dry.

The following astringent wash has proved invaluable in reducing the pitted appearance left by overlarge pores. But it must be made fresh every two days or so, for it is highly perishable and will not keep longer.

PORE REFINER

1½ ounces cucumber juice   5 ounces elder flower water
½ ounce tincture of benzoin

A bottle is easiest to use with this preparation, so pour in the mixed cucumber juice and elder flower water. Add the benzoin drop by drop and shake vigorously after each addition. Pour the well-blended liquid out over a fine cheesecloth in order to catch the unblendable particles of benzoin, then return the strained mixture to the bottle.

It is always good to keep on hand a few simple ingredients so that one is never prevented from a daily application of a refining lotion or paste to the skin plagued by large pores. A hit-or-miss schedule just won't work. With daily care, you will one day be rewarded by your mirror with a reflection of a fine-textured skin which will justify all the trouble.

Camphor is a good standby in the treatment of unsightly pores. Sprinkle a few drops in your rinse water and you can feel the tightening effect almost immediately. Only a few drops, though. Never try to make up for lost time when you undergo a special skin treatment. If a little is good, stay with it. A lot will not make a better solution, but just a stronger and probably undesirable one. Work with a minimum of ingredients until you know the reactions of your skin.

SKIN TONERS AND TIGHTENERS

In order to achieve one's finest appearance, it is not enough just to clean the face and feed the skin. For some skins will misbehave under makeup, and all that work goes for nothing. Along with learning to care for the skin, the value of an effective skin toner must be recognized.

Cucumber juice very effectively brings life to skin that rebels under makeup. Try this old French recipe and watch your skin develop tone. But remember, using it once or twice will not work. It is the consistent daily and nightly application that will produce worthwhile results.

Squeeze the juice from two cucumbers and heat to the boiling point before skimming away the froth and bottling the liquid. Keep refrigerated and use one teaspoon of the juice to two teaspoons of water. Carefully pat on the face and neck night and morning and allow to dry.

Lettuce has been used for centuries to refine the skin. Delicate creams can be made by including the strained juice of the pale green leaves into a lanolin base. But an even simpler preparation can be quickly applied directly to the skin with excellent results, if repeated often enough.

Break the stems and stalks of garden lettuce after it has reached a height permitting stalk development. Rub the milky fluid coming from the stalk over the face before retiring. Rinse off in the morning with tepid water, then cool and blot dry.

Of course, any of the vinegar toilet waters are helpful in toning and tightening the skin (see Chapter One.) You can whip up perfumed vinegars by using strawberries, raspberries, any of the family of mints or even scented herbs. They are all a delightful addition to the cosmetic shelf, for in addition to their individual qualities, they have a fresh, sharp scent that helps to disguise the acrid vinegar odor.

But if you are short on time and don't object to the smell of straight vinegar, simply use plain apple cider vinegar by pouring a dab into your final rinse.

The use of egg whites to tighten the pores and bring tone to the complexion should especially be practiced by those with the additional problem of oily skin. This is such an easy habit to acquire that no special preparations are necessary. Simply dip your fingers into the empty egg shell, after using the egg in food preparation. Catch up the remaining egg white and smooth it over your face.

There is always enough residue within an egg shell to provide daily treatment at no additional cost. Breakfast time, when there are scrambled or poached eggs on the menu, is an excellent time to use the egg-white covering. One woman found that by using the residue egg white for a beauty treatment when she prepared her family's breakfast, she was able not only to tighten facial pores, but she eliminated fine lines developing around the mouth. After breakfast she rinsed away the dried egg white and lightly oiled her face with corn oil. This was later rinsed away as she dressed for the day. By then she had given her face two beauty treatments without setting aside any extra time.

You can also keep a whole egg white in a jar with a lid in the refrigerator. Remove a teaspoon or so each time you need it.

To add nutrition to the egg white as a skin tightener, combine a tablespoon of skim milk powder to one unbeaten egg white and beat together thoroughly. This masque aids an oily skin and provides an astringent action while it feeds the skin.

Another variation of the egg-white tightener is a mixture of the juice of a few sprigs of mint and a few drops of honey with the egg white. This is allowed to dry on the face before it is rinsed away.

CHAPTER SIX

Honey, The Rejuvenator

Honey as a food was recognized as a life-sustainer even in pre-Biblical days. Cavemen learned to grab combs of honey from hidden hives, as they warded off the stings of a million angry bees, because of the life-giving and delicious properties of this amber nectar. Honey has been used both as a food and as a cosmetic throughout the centuries. As a source of quick energy because of its predigested natural sugars, honey has no equal. Easily assimilated, its vitamins and minerals boost its value as a health-giving food.

Those same vitamins and minerals turn it into a powerhouse cosmetic when a poorly nourished body produces a skin that is clogged and muddy. Repeated applications of tissue-building honey will bring a glow of color where none existed before.

In addition, honey's bacteria-destroying actions aid patches of inflamed skin. The soothing, thick liquid that heals and nourishes is one of the finest of all skin foods.

Balms, lotions and unguents using honey as a main ingredient have been found to repair sensitive skins that cannot tolerate much activity. Roughened hands dipped into vats of honey in primitive fashion lose their coarsened texture. Bit by bit the healing and beautifying properties of this wonder food were discovered and praised and put to good use.

Today we know the hygroscopic nature of honey attracts and holds moisture to the skin, thus restoring dried, aging tissue at least as long as the applications of honey are used.

Of such great value is the bee industry that all parts of honey production can be used. Beeswax itself is the basis of all good lipsticks, and if one has the proper molds, it is possible to produce a lipstick without the coal tar dyes that keep the lips of women around the world in a continual state of peeling.

Not only the wax, but pollen, carried on the tiny legs of the bees as they dip in and out of blossoms in search of sweet nectar to convert to honey, enriches the honey itself. Pollen has been called nature's richest food. It is small wonder that nutritional richness such as this brings so many beautifying and healing qualities with its use.

Of course, as with any sugar, too much honey as a food should not be consumed. For all its healthy qualities, because of its sugar content, it should be taken in moderation (and sometimes not at all—particularly by diabetics or hypoglycemics). But there is no limit to its external application, for although only a fraction is absorbed by the skin, it is enough to produce the effects we are after.

Honey can restore a more youthful appearance by the simplest dab on the face or in complicated creams and lotions. Here is a trial facial: splash warm water across a freshly washed face. Do not use any of the other applications suggested in this book, other than perhaps an astringent lotion after cleansing. Otherwise, you place a film barrier over the very pores you are trying to reach. Reserve your creams for later.

Having moistened your face, dip two fingers into a teaspoon of raw, unheated honey. In upward sweeping motions, lightly spread it into every area of your face. Be sure your hair is drawn back and your face fully exposed to the edges of the ear lobes and the top of the forehead for this facial honey bath.

Allow the honey to remain for twenty minutes before rinsing away with warm water. Daily applications of honey can refine and soften skin that has hardened from exposure or poor care. Honey is also helpful to use after removing makeup. Directly after its use, a final rinse in a mixed solution of apple cider vinegar and water will bring a further glow to the skin.

There are always means at hand to combat early wrinkles. And the glory of using one's kitchen as a beauty laboratory is that many of the needed ingredients are already there. As long as you keep a jar of raw, unheated honey on your shelf, half the battle against incipient wrinkles is won.

One quick and remedial recipe combines one teaspoon of honey with two tablespoons of sweet cream. Before milk was homogenized, you could simply lift the cream from the top of the bottle of milk. But if you don't have access to fresh, certified, raw milk, you will have to resort to buying either light cream, sometimes called coffee cream, or heavy whipping cream. Be sure that it is not a milk "food" or other substitute.

Beat the ingredients together and apply to a freshly scrubbed, rinsed and dried face. With the fingertips, pat the mixture into creases and lines.

With a gentle rubbing action, saturate the grooved lines, and as you apply the honey and cream, spread the lines on the face apart. Do not pull or work roughly. Smooth the area instead, and attempt to uncrease the lines.

This is a quickie treatment that can soften the early wrinkling areas around the eyes, mouth and on the forehead. The practice could beneficially become a morning ritual, accompanying breakfast preparation and rinsed away afterward.

Another kitchen treatment using honey with minimum preparation is to mix one-half teaspoon of apple cider vinegar or lemon juice with two tablespoons of honey. Blend together and spread over the face. Allow this to remain on for fifteen or twenty minutes before rinsing away in warm water and blotting the skin dry. This softens and deep cleans, leaving the skin refreshed and free of accumulated oils that a cleansing cream cannot reach.

These mixtures are also excellent for the neck. In fact,

this part of the body is usually in as much need of attention as the face and often neglected. One's glance simply doesn't begin and end with the face, but continues over the full expanse of both face and neck.

Honey and almonds in combination is one of the finest cosmetic teams we have. The qualities of both have long been recognized by women around the world who have mastered the art of looking their best at all times. In earlier days there was an excellent commercial preparation using the two items alone.

But more glamorous products seem to have pushed aside this simple, effective skin preserver and rejuvenator. So here is the old recipe, in all its grand simplicity. It is really like having a pot of gold on hand to have this delightful potion on your cosmetic shelf.

Buy a one-pound jar of U.S.P. lanolin (which means it is approved for pharmaceutical use). Choose the hydrous kind which does not require mixing with water. You will need one-half pound of the lanolin in the following recipe; save the remainder for other recipes.

Place one-fourth pound of raw honey in the top of a double boiler, and as it warms, beat in one-half pound of lanolin. As this melts, add one-half cup of sweet almond oil and stir until well blended.

Remove from the heat and beat thoroughly with an electric or hand beater. Get a complete emulsification and then pour into convenient-size jars. Keep all but the jar you are using in the refrigerator. Label the jars carefully so they aren't mistaken for food.

Use the cream liberally over neck, face and elbows. It still has all the magic it had when our grandmothers stepped out smelling of honey and almond cream.

Honey water as a rinse is handed down to us in various recipes. Since it has been in recorded use from the heyday of the Roman empire, there has been ample time to experiment and improve it. Nevertheless, it remains much like the original.

HONEY WATER

4 ounces honey	¼ ounce cloves
½ ounce grated lemon peel	½ ounce nutmeg
½ ounce grated orange peel	2 ounces rose water
½ ounce benzoin	2 ounces elder flower water
½ ounce storax	12 ounces ethyl alcohol

Pour the honey into a two-quart glass jar and add the lemon and orange peel, benzoin, storax, cloves and nutmeg. Stir together to blend. Add the remaining ingredients and beat together. Place a lid on the jar and shake together thoroughly. Allow the mixture to steep for three days, shaking frequently, and then filter and bottle.

This fragrant water was used daily in Roman households and comes to us through the centuries as a mixture of great merit.

Honey comes to the rescue again, after a summer's sun produces blotches of brown and red on the throat and neck. When mixed with oatmeal, it brings about a softening and clearing, since the oatmeal serves as a mild bleach. The following combination, if used nightly and rinsed away each morning, will eventually eliminate the speckled appearance that is so aging.

Mix the following items together until you have an easily spreadable paste: One ounce of honey, one teaspoon of lemon juice, two unbeaten egg whites, one-half teaspoon sweet almond oil and enough oatmeal powder to make a smooth paste. Try whirling a handful of old-fashioned oatmeal in the blender for this. Or reduce oatmeal to a powder in a nut grinder. Have the mixture moist, but not dripping when you apply it to your throat and neck.

CHAPTER SEVEN

Herbal Rebuilders

After a winter of central heating and frozen vegetables or food that is trucked in from distant areas, one's complexion begins to develop a flaky appearance that suggests the lack of vitally fresh green things in the diet. Fine lines can form around the mouth and eyes as cold winds, starchy winter foods and the absence of sunlight begin to take their toll. This is especially the time to use herbs to restore good skin tone.

There is as much variety of cosmetic benefits from herbs as there are herbs themselves. They have been used to combat oiliness, refine pores and fade freckles, eliminate sallowness and increase circulation. They fight wrinkles and moisturize a dry complexion.

They also serve to smooth roughened, abused skin and as deep pore cleansers. For some problem skins there are herbal recipes that can clear up long-standing disorders. Many of these recipes have proved themselves through successive generations of use. We know that mint stimulates sluggish skin and that yarrow reduces the oily content of the pores. It requires only an inquisitive mind and adventuresome spirit to find the herbal beauty treatment that will work for you.

No product will strengthen skin tissue as well as an herbal lotion. The lowly dandelion—roots and leaves—is an excellent inner and outer tonic and cleanser for the sallow skin. Prepare a strong tea; drink one-half cup daily for two weeks and also apply the same tea as a wash for the face.

Once you have begun using dandelion wash for a yellowed complexion, you will rejoice that your facial tea grows free on your lawn and is far simpler to prepare and use than you might have believed. To supplement this beauty plan, pick young green leaves before they develop bitterness later in the summer and use them in salad.

Aside from the nutritive value and delicious crispness of fresh dandelion leaves, they are definitely beneficial for the skin. Included in the diet, the blood-cleansing *dent de lion* (or "tooth of the lion" as the dandelion is known in France) is an excellent source of the beauty vitamins A and C, plus the minerals needed for good skin growth.

The usual method of using herbs cosmetically is to prepare a tea and either combine it with other ingredients or use the herbal infusion alone as a lotion. If you are new to the world of herbs for complexion care, begin with some of the better known plants. If you are in the country on a warm summer day, collect a handful of any variety of garden or wild mint leaves. Rinse the leaves and pour a cup of boiling water over them, cover and allow to steep until the mixture is cool. Strain out the leaves and splash the mint rinse over your entire face and neck after they have been scrubbed clean. If you live in the city, buy mint tea leaves at a health or herbal store and use the same procedure.

To achieve a tingling pickup, pour the steeped and cooled, but unstrained tea into a ice cube pan. Allow the pan sectioner to remain. When the mint ice cubes form from this pure mint liquid, rub one over a freshly washed face.

This is a refreshing treatment before retiring on a summer's night. Or it is advantageously used just before applying makeup, although of course you must blot the skin dry. The chill helps close the pores and gives the skin a smoother finish.

The pungent marigold is a valuable plant when used to make a rinse for acne conditions and in clearing up skin inflammations. Marigold petals can also be lavishly sprinkled across a salad—either fruit or vegetable—or included in any dish where their unusual taste will be appreciated. Eating flowers for pleasure and beauty is an old custom, much more in use in centuries gone by than now.

The marigold, or marsh gold, is a flower of the sun, much as is the sunflower plant. As such, it follows the movements of the sun and is believed to retain much of the sun's benefits in its multi-petaled form.

When the leaves are crushed to a moist pulp they can be applied directly to heal outbreaks on the skin. For generations women have valued the golden petals as a wash for oily complexions. To make this, drop a handful of marigold petals into a cup of boiling water and steep until the water is only warm to the touch. Crush and strain the petals out of the liquid and apply the wash generously to a freshly scrubbed, rinsed and dried face. Allow the marigold liquid to dry on the skin. Repeat as often as required.

For a nourishing skin food, add one teaspoon of the freshly macerated petals to a tablespoon of lanolin, apricot or sweet almond oil. Mash the petals and stir with a wooden spoon, or other non-metallic stirrer, while the oil heats. Allow the mixture to cool somewhat and strain out the petals. The strength of the mixture can be increased by placing another teaspoon of the flower petals in the heated and strained oil, and repeating the process until you have the potency you want.

Yarrow, from the aster family of plants, since medieval days has been the treasure of those afflicted with acne or excessively oily skin. Old recipes turn up suggesting opening the facial pores with a steaming process, and then applying warm yarrow tea for healing. Modern electric facial steamers can be used, though probably the old-fashioned compresses applied directly to the face are more effective.

After either kind of steaming, pat the face with sterile cotton dipped into a strong brew of warm yarrow tea. It contains tannic and achilleic acids and essential oils which are curative.

A great detractor to beauty is the appearance of tiny red

thread-like veins that can lace themselves across the face but seem to concentrate on the lower cheeks. Freshly squeezed parsley juice helps to halt the vein breakage by strengthening the capillary walls.

In England, broken veins are bathed in coltsfoot tea. This herb can be purchased in cut or powdered form. Make a strong tea every day and apply compresses dipped into a tepid solution.

The capillary fragility which creates the small red veins running like wheel spokes beneath the skin indicates a weakness in these blood-carrying veins. Because of the damaged walls, the fluid breaks through into the areas beyond the veins.

Attacking the problem from a dietary view, the bioflavonoids (vitamin C complex with rutin) are needed to help this condition. This means a diet should be planned that is abundant in citrus fruits, rose hips, green peppers, turnip greens, cabbage, buckwheat and parsley. Rutin is derived from buckwheat.

Besides adding these foods to your daily diet, external applications of the same foods can help the complexion subject to broken veins. Apply the raw, fresh juices singly by patting onto the skin around the affected areas. Allow to dry, and leave on as long as is convenient.

Herbs can be very helpful in softening the formation of lines on the face and neck. The steady application of liquid from steeped fennel or even the pulped plant itself can lessen fine-line wrinkling. As with any other complexion aid, one or two applications will not bring about any worthwhile results. Healing with herbs is a longer and slower process than any method using commercial preparations. But if the regime is adhered to, the rewards are there and definite.

When aging lines begin to crease the mouth and eye area, it is time to turn one's most heroic efforts toward halting them. The easily grown fennel plant can be made into a facial masque when combined with raw honey and yogurt and then applied to a clean face. The thin covering should be left on for fifteen or twenty minutes and removed—not with soap—with several rinsings in tepid water.

To improve the tone and texture of an anemic, wan complexion, wash with the juice of the stinging nettle. Hugely ignored because of its blistering sting when touched directly, the nettle plant offers an astringent rinse that is of great value.

Pick the center young leaves with gloved hands and clippers, to avoid the painful blisters. Produce a soft mash for the face by simmering the chopped leaves for five or ten minutes and allow the mash to cool somewhat before applying to the face. Curative value comes from the plant hormones and minerals.

Lime flowers are not only exquisite in appearance, but are also helpful in removing skin impurities when used as a rinse. In addition, they bleach with continued use. In both treatments warm compresses of strong lime flower tea are applied directly to the skin which is then allowed to dry unaided. Rinse with tepid water and towel the skin briskly.

Sage tea offers an excellent method for opening and cleaning clogged pores and revitalizing the tissue. As it is a rather strong astringent, it should be cautiously used. Taken internally, it aids in perspiration and assists the cleansing from within.

An herb becoming more and more popular in treating various skin ills is the comfrey plant. Herbalists have long extracted allantoin from the comfrey leaves and roots to rebuild skin growth in areas difficult to heal. Now comfrey as a healing agent has been rediscovered by modern medicine, and its qualities are being incorporated into cosmetic and medical preparations for commercial use.

It is easy enough to plant a comfrey root or two in your own garden. Or try growing one in a pot. It grows quickly and produces a mass of leaves. They die down in winter and reappear in the spring. They require frequent watering.

In many parts of the world comfrey has never fallen into

disuse. Stubborn and persistent skin troubles yield to compresses of the pulped leaf. But the method of application can differ. A tea can be made and used as a daily or nightly rinse. Or the leaves can be macerated and blended into a light oil base, or added to a night cream. A simple liquid application, at least once or twice daily, is probably the most beneficial. Add a few drops of water to the mash and squeeze through gauze to obtain the liquid. Or apply the macerated leaves directly on the area. The moisture left on the skin will be sufficient if applied often enough.

Aloe vera is another cosmetic plant that can be used to bring about a normal, functioning skin. Of ancient cultivation, the aloe vera has been used extensively for the treatment of body burns. The soothing application of the leaf which contains vitamins A and D, plus chlorophyll, can heal severe burns and more direct body burns without scarring.

Just as with the comfrey plant, the pure extract of juice should be used for application to body areas. However, there is more liquid in the aloe vera than in the comfrey, whose leaf produces a thick mucilaginous liquid after maceration.

The extracted aloe vera juice can also be combined with a lanolin base cream for added benefit. The moisturizing properties of the juice and the enriching lanolin soften dry, rough skin.

CHAPTER EIGHT

Facial Masques

Kitchen chemistry can provide some of the most exciting and effective skin foods imaginable for the woman who wants maximum benefit for her complexion with minimum cost and effort. The application of facial masques made from wholesome, nourishing foods is a practical means of adding easy beauty.

Different nutritional facial masques produce a variety of results. Some masques can be planned for aiding dry or oily skin, some for adding moisture to the complexion and others for lessening premature wrinkling and aiding in the removal of blackheads and clogged pores. In fact, a suitable and well-chosen facial masque applied when needed will bring tone to the skin and protect a complexion from many problems.

When used regularly, facial masques can make the skin glow with vitality and remove years from one's appearance.

It is not wise to depend on the average diet for a good skin condition. There are too many assaults made upon it from valueless foods, pollution of both air and water and daily applications of chemicalized makeup. In time, even the most robust of skins will rebel. However, the stimulation of facial masques brings needed circulation to every pore on the face and revitalizes the skin. Masques are not a luxury, but a necessity for proper skin care.

Nature offers a bountiful supply of beauty products for use in masques. Not only fruits and vegetables are excellent sources, but yogurt, brewer's yeast and fuller's earth have practical purposes, too. Eggs, mayonnaise, and oils mixed with wheat germ provide good nutrition and are anti-wrinkling in their richness.

For clearing away accumulated tissue debris, the ripened papaya fruit does an almost miraculous job. Literally eating away the dead cells that pile up to dull the complexion, the mashed papaya rejuvenates the fresh skin lying concealed beneath the old.

When using the papaya or any fruit in a masque, you must lie down to keep it on your face.

Apply the mashed papaya to all areas of the face except around the eyes. Allow the pulp to remain on for fifteen to twenty minutes before rinsing away. Try the papaya twice a week until your skin feels fresh and alive, and any surface flakiness has disappeared.

Those who have most benefited from this facial declare that whenever practical, the papaya should be eaten as well as used as a masque. The powerful papain enzyme contained in papaya pulp breaks down the protein in the diet and prepares it for easier assimilation. This helps to prevent the muddy complexion caused by faulty digestion and poor elimination.

Another cleansing fruit, which also bleaches, is the sun-ripened strawberry. Strawberries have long been used by women seeking to restore their complexions to a smooth, youthful condition. These berries will really accomplish this if you persist in the application. They are also an excellent carrier for other skin foods. They can be crushed and mixed with oatmeal, cream, plain water or used alone, according to your special need.

Beauties of long ago relied heavily on the strawberry for softening and bleaching. Genevieve, a friend who lived in North Africa for many years and yet retained her exquisite moon-glow complexion, attributes this to her frequent use of strawberry mash. The berries must be vine ripened to be most effective. Select juicy, plump berries, rinse and shake dry. Crush them with a silver fork and spread over a freshly scrubbed face. Rinse after fifteen or twenty minutes with tepid water and pat dry. This can be used on successive days until the skin is smooth and clear. If the skin proves sensitive to this treatment, apply salad oil afterward, and blot off or dilute the mash with a little water before using.

The combination of strawberries mashed with cream offers a vitamin feast for the skin. Vitamins A and C are also skin vitamins, and this masque which contains both can cleanse and stimulate dull skin miraculously.

Ripened pears offer an astringent action to the oily skin and the fruit also contains a disinfectant. Teenagers with skin outbreaks should especially profit from this masque.

Watermelon juice provides a strengthening wash that is also helpful in removing tiny, surface wrinkles. An excellent source of Vitamin A and C, it will relieve dry, horny skin if used daily during the summer months. This naturally distilled fruit water also deep-cleanses and tightens the pores. Again, for additional value, eat the melon frequently as well.

One of the most practical of fruit treatments comes from grapes. They are easy to keep on hand in small bunches, and several a day would suffice for a refreshing, skin-tightening facial masque. Grind a handful of emerald green grapes in your blender until they are pulpy.

When there isn't time to lie down, you can snatch in-between pick-ups by biting off a grape tip and scouring the face from top to bottom with it. While green grapes offer a refreshing feeling with their light, sweet nectar, any grape will be effective on the skin. Some people believe that green grapes should be used on dry skin and red grapes on oily skin. A normal skin can profit from using either.

Facial masques offer such great variety of benefits to your complexion. With abundant fruits to be had the year round, you can change about as you wish, bringing the different qualities of each fruit to a needy skin. The same thing is true of vegetable masques which are equally important. Either or both should be used the year round.

Winter is a wonderful time to try a cabbage juice facial, made from the pure juice of a few green leaves of cabbage.

Use a juicer as the easiest means of extracting cabbage juice. Or try a grater, squeezing the ground cabbage through cheesecloth in order to get a teaspoon or two of the liquid. Pat this into the skin and allow it to dry on and remain as long as possible. This fine skin toner brings a lustre to pale skin and is particularly beneficial to oily skin. The sulphur and chlorine content in the outer green leaves cleanses and purifies. Cabbage juice is a splendid skin tightener, producing a youthful, fresh appearance as it pulls sagging skin together.

With all of these masques, benefits increase with the number of applications. One facial masque may be refreshing, but it will take many to bring real results. Just as one good, balanced meal a week could not equal the effect of daily balanced meals, neither can a quickie facial have the lasting effects of frequent masques.

Cucumber masques have been used to refine, clean and bleach skins for centuries. Even in medieval times, maidens were known to be partial to the cooling, refreshing qualities of cucumber when it was squeezed and applied to the skin, or when more elaborate preparations were made combining it with unguents, creams and even mutton fat. In the sixteenth century, cucumber was popular both as a food and as a complexion wash for clearing up "fierie noses, pimples, pumples, rubis, and such like."

Today's modern cosmetics are liberally laced with cucumber extract for the same reasons. But it is easy enough to skip the cream base and apply fresh cucumber directly to the skin for impressive results.

For a solid masque, grind or mash thoroughly enough cucumber to cover the face, and after a restful twenty minutes or more, rinse away and pat dry. As a mid-day refresher, either masque or juice stimulates the skin.

Complexion needs are greater in winter, for it is then that one can lose tone and color and develop a greyness that defies every pot of cream on your shelf.

Facial Masques

While creams certainly play an important role in maintaining a good skin condition, they cannot bring color or freshness to the skin as efficiently as masques made from foods and used regularly.

When winter has whipped the skin dry, a brewer's yeast masque can restore rosiness. An invigorating treatment, the yeast masque pulls the pores together and brings a surge of fresh blood to help nourish the skin. This protein-packed food should also be taken internally. Brewer's yeast, one of the greatest beauty foods, can even eliminate the use for blushers and rouge if used in sufficient quantity, and often enough.

Prepare an easily spreadable paste of one teaspoon of powdered, grain-grown brewer's yeast and two teaspoons of warm water. Mineral water is best, but any water will do. Adjust the consistency with additional water if necessary, but do not make it thin enough to drip from the face. Apply the mixture to a freshly scrubbed face and pat in briskly with the fingertips.

Whereas most of the other masques suggested are soothing and healing in application, a brewer's yeast masque draws a fresh blood supply to underlying areas and produces a pulling or tautening sensation. This is really a self-massage of the skin, and pores are nourished and stimulated by this very practical and efficient masque.

Such a masque has to be timed individually. Some skins profit from thirty minutes which might be too long for more sensitive complexions. Aim for fifteen to twenty minutes in the beginning and extend the time as desired. The skin should surge with color, and after the masque is removed with a fresh washcloth and warm water, your face will feel satiny.

Although this masque particularly helps oily skins, any skin condition should profit from its application. For dry skin add a teaspoon of wheat germ or other vegetable or nut oil in place of one of water. Or after using the brewer's yeast masque, apply a thin coating of salad oil to the cleansed face.

Wheat germ and egg yolk, thinned to a paste with a few drops of milk, is another very good masque. You are feeding your face with class A protein in the egg which is rich in every vitamin except C, plus all the important minerals. Wheat germ contributes vitamin E, the milk, vitamin D. Spread this beauty cocktail on the face frequently to nourish dry skin and prevent wrinkles.

The more careful you are of the freshness of your foods, for internal or external use, the more benefits your skin will reap. If the eggs are fertile, you are adding additional vitamin E to your skin. Avoid toasted wheat germ in all preparations. Choose instead the plain, raw germ. Milk of course, if raw and certified, will bring assimilable calcium and vitamin D.

To remove these thicker masques which harden somewhat on the skin, use a washcloth dipped in warm water.

Getting down to the very earth itself for materials for beauty, fuller's earth is a convenient powder that keeps well and is always available for a reviving masque that does much the same work as brewer's yeast, but without the same amount of nourishment. However, as a pure substance of the earth, it has its quota of minerals plus its ability to step up the circulation in a sluggish complexion. The earth masque slowly hardens as it dries, but stimulates the bloodstream which carries away impurities and quickens dull circulation.

Mix only small quantities of any masque at a time. A fuller's earth masque slides like satin onto the face and complete coverage requires only one tablespoon of the earth to one tablespoon of warm water. It should remain on until completely dry. Depending upon the consistency, this could be from fifteen to thirty minutes. Don't rush the procedure. Rinse away with warm water. The skin will glow after its removal. But don't use this masque too often as it is of a drying nature. A thin coating of salad oil is helpful after rinsing away the masque.

An oatmeal masque offers untold rewards to a blotchy,

aging appearance when employed on an every-other-day basis. There is something almost uncanny about the potency of oatmeal, used both as an internal food and as a skin food, particularly when applied in the form of a masque.

Add two tablespoons of old-fashioned oatmeal to one-half cup of milk and cook to a soft consistency. Add two teaspoons of elder flower, orange or rose water. Beat together and when barely warm, spread over the face and neck. Leave this on for twenty minutes before rinsing away and blotting dry.

For rejuvenating a parchment-like complexion, there is no more effective masque than a combination of egg yolk and oil. Beat together the yolk of an egg with one-half teaspoon of wheat germ, apricot, sweet almond, corn or olive oil. Add a few drops of mineral water and beat again. Using an artist's brush, paint this mixture on the face and throat and neck. As it begins to dry, brush on a second coat and lie on a slant board for twenty minutes. The rich and potent food values of the egg and oil penetrate thirsty skin, and the twenty-minute saturation brings renewed life.

CHAPTER NINE

Lotions and Potions

Lotions moisturize the skin in a most pleasant and effective manner. In addition, according to the ingredients used, they can also soften, bleach, cleanse, feed and heal. The proper use of these lotions is very often an acquired beauty habit. Many women feel that all they really need to do is to clean the skin and concentrate on some specific complexion problem.

But lotions are often the neglected performers of many unrealized benefits. Herbs, nuts, seeds, grasses and flowers can be made into solutions that improve even the finest skins. These liquids are quickly absorbed, easily blending into the skin.

They are convenient to use because they can be dabbed on any time. When you are free for a moment, and your face is without makeup and clean, pat on a lotion and forget about having to remove it later.

It will pay off in huge dividends. Many times the nutrition in a skin lotion can supply just the needed ingredient for a blooming complexion. So lotions are more than simply emollients or refreshers.

While any time of the day is a good time to use a skin lotion, an overnight application allows a slower, longer time for penetration and absorption, and brings the delight of awakening in the morning with a visibly improved skin. Remember, maximum beauty is possible only when maximum skin care is provided. One can get by without the extras in a beauty program, but it is not the wisest way.

A treasured recipe for smoothing roughened skin comes from the file of a beautician who lived nearly a century ago.

If your source of fresh bean blossoms is as organic and fresh as Harriet Hubbard Ayer's, you should have the same exquisite results that caused her to count this as one of her favorite lotions.

This charming bean flower lotion is said to have contributed to the finest of complexions in the days when a woman wanted pearly skin tones touched with a tint of natural roses. The recipe sounds like a Chinese poem.

BEAN FLOWER LOTION

¼ pound bean flowers
1½ ounce rose petals
1 cup distilled water
the juice of ½ lemon

Mix together the first three ingredients and distill in a water bath (as suggested in Chapter Two) until about a cup of liquid is produced. Add the juice of one-half lemon and beat together. Keep the liquid tightly corked and apply to the face each evening and morning, allowing the fragrant liquid to dry on the skin. Only a small amount is required, as it should not drip from the face during application.

Hungary water was highly regarded and used long ago. A monk is supposed to have presented the coveted recipe to Queen Elisabeth of Hungary in the fourteenth century, making this the first known toilet water which was prepared with alcohol spirits. The queen, whose beauty endured well into her seventies, attributed her striking appearance to this lotion. Other accounts say that although Queen Elisabeth was a beautiful woman concerned with maintaining her appearance, she did not use Hungary water as a cosmetic, but as a stimulating lotion for her lameness.

Whatever the real story, the lotion has been regarded highly enough to survive some five centuries of preparation and enjoyment by women around the world.

Although the original recipe incorporated mainly rosemary leaves distilled in alcohol with lavender flowers or lemon added on occasion, there have been many interpretations. An easy version calls for one-half cup of fresh rosemary leaves, one teaspoon of grated orange peel, one grated nutmeg, one teaspoon of ground cinnamon and one handful of fresh mint leaves.

Macerate the leaves and spices and pour over them one quart of ethyl alcohol. Place in a glass jar with a lid and allow to steep for two weeks. Filter the liquid and bottle. Use for refreshing the entire body and bathing away oily residues.

The French women have always been great users of floral and herbal lotions. Each family has its own favored *tonique* or lotion. An old formula, French milk of roses, was so popular that it reached this country by the middle of the eighteen hundreds and became a national favorite.

MILK OF ROSES

1¼ pints of rose water
½ cup of rosemary water
1 ounce tincture of benzoin
1 ounce tincture of storax
¼ ounce esprit de rose

Mix together the rose water and rosemary water. Beat in the benzoin drop by drop, followed by the storax. Perfume with esprit de rose. Use twice a day, or as desired, as a complexion wash for softening reddened and chapped skin. As a substitute for the once easily obtained esprit de rose, simply add a drop or two of oil of roses, or any perfume, and blend.

Benzoin is often used in complexion washes and lotions because of its stimulating resin from balsam. Its aromatic scent brings a freshness of the outdoors, and its resinous qualities heal and soothe an irritated skin. If left on the skin overnight, it strengthens the skin tissue itself. Minor complexion flare-ups will be notably lessened after an application of a wash containing a few drops of benzoin. One caution: clean the top of the benzoin bottle carefully before replacing or it will stick.

Virgin's milk is an effective benzoin lotion. Easy to make, it can be kept on hand to use when an unsightly blemish suddenly appears and must be dealt with immediately. To make this lotion, place one cup of rose water in a bottle and add 1 teaspoon of tincture of benzoin drop by drop, shaking vigorously each time.

Though the old recipes usually specified rose water as the basis for virgin's milk, it works equally well with elder flower water or orange water.

For the skin that reacts unfavorably even to mild exposure to sun and wind, special attention must be given to prevent chronic chafing and flaking. Usually this condition does not exist when the diet is adequate (see Chapter Thirteen.) But when a poor diet results in overly sensitive skin, the problem should be attacked both from within and without.

Sometimes a soothing oil can be worked into the skin to give protection. The following lotion is an additional help.

Combine one-fourth cup of fresh cucumber juice, one-half cup of rose water, one-fourth cup of elder flower water and one-fourth teaspoon of ethyl alcohol. Shake together in a covered glass jar to blend. Now add, drop by drop, in order to mix well, fifteen drops of tincture of benzoin. Shake vigorously after each drop of benzoin.

Apply once or twice a day to prevent or counter roughened and irritated skin. The healing, soothing qualities of this lotion would make it a favorite, and it is easily made.

We have already learned that applying fresh vegetables and fruits to the skin can nourish and cleanse it. But often there is just not enough time to relax with a fresh masque. Then it is always good to have a complexion lotion on hand. Our old friend the cucumber, made into a milk lotion, offers a splendid pick-up for end-of-the-day complexion fatigue. The following is a simplified version of an ancient recipe.

Mince one cucumber fine, place it in a glass pot and cover it with one-third cup of boiling water. Place a lid on the pot to prevent evaporation and simmer over very low heat for thirty minutes. Watch carefully to prevent complete loss of water or scorching.

Strain the mixture into a bowl and add enough tincture

of benzoin, drop by drop, to give the liquid a milky appearance. Beat continuously to insure complete blending. Add one-third cup of boiling water to the mixture and beat thoroughly again.

Milk lotions require emulsification in order to prevent a separation in the bottle after they have been prepared. In commercial cosmetics, this is accomplished by the addition of waxes, soaps and other items. By preparing your own personal lotions, you avoid using these unnecessary preservatives on your skin.

An egg beater used with vigor, if the quantity is large enough, will usually blend the ingredients properly. If separation does occur, merely shake the contents vigorously to blend again.

MILK OF ALMONDS

Place one ounce of freshly shelled sweet almonds in a strainer and dip alternately into boiling and cold water. As soon as the skins soften enough, slip them off the almonds and place the blanched almonds on paper towelling to dry. Grind the dried almonds in a mortar with a pestle until a powder is produced. Add one-half pint of distilled water, pouring it in a few drops at a time. Grind the nut powder until you have a smooth, milky liquid.

Strain this emulsion through a piece of gauze to remove any coarse particles.

Another skin lotion is appealing if only because its users are famous the world over for their incredibly lovely complexions. English milk of roses sounds as pretty as it is useful. And English women endorse it enthusiastically. One seldom sees the roughened, dried complexions in England that are found elsewhere in the world.

While the moist climate probably is conducive to that fresh English look, indifferent care can still ruin it. The younger generation has turned, in great part, to the commercial preparations that are used elsewhere. Therefore, English women now in their fifties and sixties can easily compete with younger women in the delicacy of their skins.

ENGLISH MILK OF ROSES

Grind one and one-half ounces of freshly shelled and blanched almonds in a mortar, bowl or grinder. After producing a finely ground powder, add three-fourths of a pint of rose water, pouring slowly enough to permit a complete blending. Stir in one-half teaspoon of finely powdered castile soap and one-half teaspoon of sweet almond oil. Beat the mixture with an egg beater until it is completely emulsified.

Mix in a separate bowl two and one-half ounces of ethyl alcohol with one-fourth teaspoonful of essence of roses. Add enough rose water to make one pint of liquid. Stir the second mixture into the first and continue to beat until the mixtures are completely blended.

From our own land comes a refreshing lotion that can cool a heated skin on the warmest day and still produce a glowing complexion. Lettuce milk is considered a standby for blotchy flare-ups. The balm-like liquid locked within the leaves and stalks of all lettuces except iceberg, helps to hold the tissue moisture within the skin.

LETTUCE MILK

Carefully wash and dry the outer leaves of a firm head of lettuce. Boston, Bibb, or any of the homegrown varieties produce an excellent lettuce milk. Place the clean leaves in an enamel, stainless steel or glass saucepan and cover with boiling water. Place a lid on the pot and simmer the lettuce leaves for half an hour. Pour into a blender and beat until the mixture is liquified. Strain into a clean jar and add enough tincture of benzoin, one drop at a time, to create a milky appearance. Only a few drops are needed.

Witch hazel is a greatly overlooked cosmetic boon. At one time it was used in lotions for massage, baths for tired bodies and aching feet, backs and blotchy skins. The cooling qualities of an infusion of the bark of the witch hazel shrub is a comforting summer liquid to have on hand.

Used alone, witch hazel has a soothing effect. Additional benefits can be derived from combining it with other ingredients. A pleasant face lotion with astringent qualities requires one-fourth cup of witch hazel, one-half cup of elder flower water, one-fourth cup of mint water (made from simmering a handful of peppermint leaves in water to cover, and then straining), one teaspoon of raw honey and one teaspoon of apple cider vinegar.

All the ingredients are mixed together thoroughly and used for sagging skin—and morale. Even if temporary, the uplift of this pungent lotion refreshes both mind and complexion.

Oatmeal is as effective an ingredient in a face wash as it is in a masque or a soothing bath. The wash acts as a bleach and skin softener, bringing a luster to the skin if left on for a long enough period.

In order to release the high mineral and vitamin content of oatmeal for the complexion, place one cup of old-fashioned, non-instant oatmeal in the top of a double boiler. Add a pint of water and cook over boiling water until a clear liquid forms. Strain the clear liquid through a cloth, bring to a boil again, and strain a second time.

Add enough rose water or elder flower water to produce a liquid of the consistency of milk. You may add a few drops of perfume if you like, but the combination of oatmeal liquid and rose water is pleasant by itself.

CHAPTER TEN

Hair: How to Grow It, Color It and Keep It

These days, hair is often used as a means of self-expression as well as a protection for the head worn as attractively as possible. It has also served to symbolize honor or dishonor. When France was freed of German occupation after World War II, the French people used the vital importance of hair to punish the village girls who had consorted with the enemy.

Girls who had been stunningly beautiful were marched through the village streets with their heads freshly shaved right down to the scalp. It was a shocking spectacle. All their loveliness had disappeared, and the onlookers saw instead only their naked heads. If baldness were the custom, this would have been no punishment. But in our culture hair is absolutely essential.

To grow an abundant head of hair shining with health and life, attention must be given to the source of its growth. And that does not begin with the scalp or even the individual follicle from which each strand grows.

While texture may be dictated by heredity, the bloodstream determines to a large degree the strength and condition of the hair. However, in spite of even the poorest inheritance, hair can be improved by careful external attention and a diet aimed at supplying the necessary nutrients for good hair growth.

Just as the skin reflects one's internal condition, the hair also indicates general health. Especially for those who were not fortunate enough to be born with a luxuriant mass of hair. And even if the diet includes enough of the materials required for good growth and maintenance, additional help is needed from the outside.

Because the hair is the last part of the body to receive nourishment from the bloodstream, one is taught in the practice of yoga to stand on one's head. While this position has a calming effect, it is also stimulating, for when the head is down, the brain—and the hair—receives an abundant, nourishing supply of blood.

One can begin life with thick hair but, through abuse, end up with scanty growth. On the other hand, skimpy, thin hair can be coaxed into life through a complete hair-care program.

We have all seen people with magnificent hair who lead lives completely opposed to good health practices. Indifferent diets, alcohol, smoking and no exercise do not seem to affect them. But these people are usually coasting on inherited traits, and eventually destructive habits will catch up with them. Early or patchy baldness, receding hairline, dry, brittle hair and fading are the frequent results.

However, for those who have inherited that fine baby-like hair so difficult to manage, there is definite hope.

The first step is a complete evaluation of hair condition and living habits. Is your hair fine? Thin? Skimpy? Slow-growing? Oily? Dry? Lackluster?

Having defined the state and condition of your hair, look into your personal habits and list them. Insufficient sleep? Tendency toward nervousness? No regular exercise? Frequent shampoos of a quick soaping and rinsing under the shower? What about your diet? List a full day's intake of food including beverages and snacks.

With all the facts neatly at hand, you are now in a position to take steps. It is of little value to run from one remedy to another or to try a new product on the hard-selling market and expect good results. Many times with such actions you merely compound your difficulties.

It is far better to aid difficult hair by an individualized

approach. Of course, medical needs should not be ignored. But after you are familiar with the requirements for good hair growth and good nutrition, a personal interest and dedicated care-plan can make the most recalcitrant hair healthy.

Many hair problems can be overcome by developing the body, or substance, of the hair. This is not as difficult as it may seem; it can be resolved by an internal and an external plan. Diet is the first consideration, and since a sufficient supply of the vitamins and minerals necessary for hair growth insures an overall improvement, the results are altogether beneficial.

Look over your list of food intake and check off useless items. These include all foods with sugar and all empty carbohydrates. Breads, rolls, pastries, gravies, cream dishes, packaged foods, soft drinks, and coffee and tea overload the average diet.

Now draw up a new list from which you will choose abundant proteins to feed your hair. Include fish, eggs, cheese and organ meats. Add whole grain cereals, such as old-fashioned oatmeal, buckwheat, brown rice, cornmeal and wheat germ. Vegetables should be fresh and used either raw or lightly steamed. Fruit should be fresh, never canned. Nut meats, fresh from their shells, sunflower and other seeds, in addition to brewer's yeast, are all rich in nutrients required for good hair growth.

A daily salad of raw vegetables should be liberally laced with a cold-pressed salad oil and apple cider vinegar. (See Chapter Thirteen.) This diet will, if adhered to, eliminate a major cause of hair problems, even as it encourages new life and develops tone to the hair. For people particularly concerned with losing hair, diet must be considered as the major redeemer.

There are other corrective dietary measures for problems. For oily, lank hair conditions, elimination of large amounts of animal fats, including bacon, butter, lard and fatty meat, will correct the over-secretion from the oil glands in the scalp. And dry, brittle hair can become silky and manageable with the addition of ample vegetable or nut oils in the diet. A daily intake of one to two tablespoons of unrefined salad oil has been known to correct the most unattractive flyaway hair. If you are using your oil on a salad, then be sure to drink the remaining bit in the bowl, for much of the oil will find its way there instead of on the salad greens.

Another help for dry hair is a hot oil treatment twice a month or as often as needed. Warm two tablespoons of olive oil or any other salad oil over hot water until it is comfortable to the touch. Gently massage this into every part of the scalp. Wring out a towel in hot water and wind it turban style around the head. As it cools, repeat the process two or three times to insure total saturation of the hair. Shampoo thoroughly and rinse, adding two tablespoons of apple cider vinegar to the last rinse water for brunettes and the same amount of lemon juice for blondes.

This beneficial hot-oil treatment restores life to straw-like hair. While the method should not exclude the search for the real cause of dry hair, it will keep damaged hair from breaking.

Another treatment for strengthening water-weakened or fragile hair is to apply castor oil, combing it thoroughly through the hair to insure complete distribution. Place a plastic bag over the hair, tucking under the edges to permit the scalp heat to aid in penetration. This thick oil is about the finest external aid possible for weakened hair. A monthly treatment is good insurance for such hair problems. Afterward, two thorough herbal shampoos are necessary, followed by a rinse with two tablespoons of apple cider vinegar or lemon juice in the last water.

If you have dark hair, and want to keep it shining and lustrous, try the formula used by Queen Anne of England. This is not a treatment for those with light or blonde hair, for it has a definite darkening quality.

To make the formula that pleased a queen, pour one-half

cup of cold-pressed green olive oil and one cup of honey into a glass jar. Stir together and then place a lid on the jar and shake vigorously. Allow the mixture to steep for a day or two before using and do not refrigerate.

Queen Anne's formula would be used prior to a shampoo. Give the jar and its contents a good shaking before use, for it separates on standing. After sectioning off the hair, apply the liquid to every part of the scalp. Rub in briskly, massaging the scalp thoroughly.

Now concentrate on the hair itself, and apply a liberal amount of the honey and oil mixture as you work your fingertips through. For complete distribution, finally comb or brush the hair without touching the scalp.

Place a plastic bag over the hair and tuck in the ends to make it airtight, while you relax for thirty minutes. Now you are ready for a stimulating shampoo that will remove all of the liquid that hasn't soaked into the hair and scalp.

Shampoo twice, scrubbing and rinsing well to be sure there is no residue oiliness. In the final rinse water, add a little apple cider vinegar or lemon juice, which will remove the last bit of soap.

This shampoo treatment has found favor with many, and its benefits increase with use. Dry, dull and lifeless hair begins to take on a new gloss with one or two monthly dousings. The frequency of use must be an individual decision. It can be used every other week, with regular shampoos in between; sometimes once a month is all that is needed.

The egg-yolk shampoo was known as a conditioner long before the term became commercially popular. Total saturation of the hair with a mixture of egg yolk and warm water can put a bounce in limp hair. It can also give superb sheen, rid the scalp of dandruff, strengthen the hair and nourish the scalp.

The egg shampoo must be one of the wonder applications of all times. There are many worthwhile formulas for hair care, but the high protein content of an egg yolk seems to be the panacea for problem hair. Old homemaker formulas list the egg shampoo as a treatment for all manner of hair difficulties. It not only cures, but if used as a maintenance shampoo, it will also prevent a recurrence of the problem.

In its most simple, pure form, two egg yolks are beaten thoroughly into a cup of warm water. This is carefully massaged into both scalp and hair. And here is the secret. A quick wash with an egg shampoo will *not* bring results. You must massage for five minutes and then soak, thoroughly saturating the hair strands and scalp.

The egg must have time to be absorbed to the fullest degree. You are actually feeding your hair protein. At the same time the egg cleans and conditions. A plastic bag placed over the scalp for at least five minutes expedites the job. After complete saturation, rinse the hair with a spray attachment if possible. This makes the removal of the egg easier, for rinsing is also a vital part of the treatment. The hair *must* be thoroughly rinsed, or the shampoo is ineffective.

For thin or short hair, one egg yolk mixed with one-half cup of water will probably produce sufficient shampoo. For a medium thick head of hair, mix two egg yolks with one cup of water and use three egg yolks for thick hair.

There are probably dozens of interesting variations of the egg-yolk shampoo. One of them includes brandy in place of one-half of the water mixture. But remember, no soap is used either before or after this marvelous egg shampoo.

Any shampoo should be chosen very carefully. A harsh shampoo can increase, rather than alleviate, problems. Shampoos should not strip the hair of its vital oils but remove accumulations of dust and oil. The frequency of shampoos should be dictated by need rather than rule. Oily hair conditions should be corrected from within; but, at the same time, oily hair requires more washing than dry hair.

Herbal shampoos supply an antiseptic action without resorting to harsh cleansers. A strong tea made of rosemary and added to a castile shampoo stimulates hair growth.

Tender nettle leaves simmered until soft and then strained, will produce a liquid that will improve hair coloring and give it body. However, as we have said before, beware the stinging nettle. Remember that the leaves possess a formic acid liquid which will raise painful blisters on the skin. Use gloves and scissors to gather the top clusters of leaves and drop them into boiling water to render them harmless and useful.

To prepare your own organic shampoo, use two ounces of soapbark chips to one pint of water. Simmer together until the liquid is reduced by one-half. A few drops of oil of rosemary give additional benefits. Strain and use as a shampoo. Soapbark is available through botanical suppliers.

The trees and fields in rural areas have always yielded their wealth to people knowledgeable in folkways. A tea made from willow bark gathered in the springtime and massaged into the hair and scalp before a regular shampoo acts as an astringent on oily hair. So rich are the properties of the willow tree that it has been used for centuries to clear up dandruff. There are other dandruff destroyers, such as one part apple juice to three parts of water rubbed into the scalp two or three times weekly. And grated burdock root, rosemary, sage and thyme simmered together in water for a few minutes and strained. A teaspoon of each of these dried herbs dropped into a pint of water yields the needed strength. Use undiluted as your final rinse after a shampoo.

One recipe for conditioning that varies but little from one country to another calls for one teaspoon each of grated burdock root, southernwood and rosemary in one cup of olive or sweet almond oil. Heat in the sun in a closed container for a week. Then rub the oil thoroughly into the roots of the hair half an hour before shampooing.

Raspberry leaves made into a strong tea and used in the final rinse water acts as a disinfectant and normalizer, producing a natural acid scalp condition.

A combination of brushing and dry shampoo improves

over-washed hair or oily hair that returns to its lank condition immediately following a regular shampoo. The dry shampoo can also clean the hair without the rigors of a regular shampoo.

Cornmeal, used also for cleaning furs, can be sprinkled through the hair and brushed out, taking with it excess oils and dust. It would be wise to stand in the bathtub or outdoors to do this to avoid having cornmeal underfoot.

Another dry shampoo calls for four ounces of powdered orris root mixed with one ounce of unscented talcum powder (available from a pharmacy) sprinkled through the hair. Allow it to remain on for ten or fifteen minutes and then begin brushing. Brush steadily until the hair is free from the fine powder. A slight residue may remain from this powdery treatment, so it should be used as an emergency shampoo preceding a regular shampoo only by a day or so.

When there were fewer cures on the market for scalp and hair ailments, the hairbrush served a greater purpose and probably prevented many hair problems from arising. But with the advent of the commercial pomades, lotions, ointments and medicated shampoos that promise everything, the hairbrush began to lose ground. It now seems easier to get a quick gloss with lacquer spray than with the proverbial one hundred brush strokes.

But, properly used, the brush cleans the scalp and hair and lessens the need for frequent shampoos. Many people erroneously believe that brushing increases the oil flow from the sebaceous glands. Actually, brushing brings up only the oil that has already been exuded and is clogging the lower portion of the hair strands and the scalp. The stimulating action of daily brushing carries the natural oil flow to the ends of the hair.

Dandruff can sometimes be avoided and even cured by the daily use of a firm, natural-bristle brush. Avoid using nylon brushes on the scalp. The inflexible nylon is irritating and can even create balding areas by its harsh scratching.

Severe hair breakage, thinning and loss of hair can result from too frequent use of plastic rollers, pincurls and the hair dryer. All of these hair-helps should be used in moderation.

Bleaching and stripping weaken and possibly destroy normal, healthy hair. If the hair structure is basically strong, damage takes longer to become apparent. But sooner or later severe methods used to remove color from the hair will destroy easy hair growth. Dry, dull and lifeless hair will have to be coaxed into a wave and eventually will not wave at all because it becomes so porous.

Special attention should be given hair that has been subjected to bleaches and chemical dyes. A protein shampoo, or an egg beaten into a mild castile shampoo, are helpful to chemically lightened hair.

The hot oil treatment and the castor oil steaming also help to offset the harshness of the stripping process. Excessively harsh bleaching procedures may offer an aesthetic value in bright tones but are hardly worth the damage and destruction they can eventually bring about. Home bleach devotees can sometimes destroy their hair in one attempt to change it overnight from a dark color to an ash or platinum shade. In the hands of an amateur, a bottle of peroxide can become a lethal weapon to the scalp and hair growth.

And more than one woman has insisted upon stripping and dyeing her own hair without reading directions carefully and has given herself a permanent immediately following the bleaching. The results of adding chemical heat to chemically saturated hair results in burnt hair with such serious breakage that sometimes it defies rehabilitation.

There are ways of changing hair color without resorting to chemical dyes, ammonia and hydrogen peroxide. Vegetable dyes and rinses are usually quite harmless, unless you have an allergy to a specific plant. This would be rare in the herbal field, but the possibility should be noted.

Of course there is no vegetable plant dye that will turn dark hair an ash blonde shade. But there are coloring agents that can tone out greying hair and bring color to fading, mousy tones. There are also ways to create lights and gloss in blonde hair which has darkened.

Vegetable plant dyes are not permanent and usually must be applied after each shampoo. However, that depends upon the hair itself, and sometimes a particular type of hair will so effectively absorb the dye that only a monthly treatment is required, except for new growth at the scalp.

In choosing a specific plant dye for your hair, select a color that most closely resembles that of your original hair coloring. Nature never creates a conflicting color scheme for us, therefore you should not attempt to lighten your hair if you have dark skin tones nor develop red hair over a sallow or olive complexion. Study your own coloring and work as closely as possible toward restoring it if you want to experiment with vegetable or plant dyes.

With the increased interest in things natural, there is now available commercially a considerable range of vegetable coloring agents considered safe for the hair. Many health food markets carry a generous color selection made from natural plant sources.

But if you want to experiment on your own, though the procedure requires some effort, you can mix your own coloring agents and come up with pleasing results.

To restore light tones to blonde hair that has lost its brilliance, a camomile solution will develop lovely new lights. These pretty little flowers can be brewed into a strong solution by mixing a cup of the dried camomile flowers with a pint of boiling water. Simmer for twenty-five minutes over a very low heat. When the liquid is cool, strain it and pour through the hair after a shampoo as the final rinse. Use a basin to catch the rinse water and repeat the procedure several times.

This rinse not only returns long-lost highlights to drab blonde hair, but acts as a tonic to both hair and scalp. The resinous oil in this attractive plant also soothes and heals an irritated scalp while it adds beauty.

Coloring the hair with a herbal rinse sometimes strengthens it, even as a deeper color tone is gained. Sage offers color and increased life to the hair. It also disposes of dandruff. A strong brew of sage and black tea creates a rich brown tone in greying hair if continued over a period of time.

Two tablespoons of black tea and two tablespoons of dried sage simmered in one quart of water for twenty-five minutes, steeped for several hours and strained, will produce a strong herbal dye. In order to be effective, this coloring agent must be massaged into hair every day until the color tone deepens to the desired shade. Once the color is satisfactory, apply only as needed. Fresh weekly preparations of the tea are necessary, however.

It is important to remember that more than one application of plant dyes is required for the most beneficial results. Color must accumulate. Vegetable dyes work very slowly, and patience is necessary to use them.

The hulls of walnuts and butternuts have been used to produce darker hair coloring. They are not easy to use as they stain not only the hair but the scalp as well. But if you care to try, take the fresh hulls from black walnuts and, handling them with gloves, drop them into boiling water. Reduce the liquid to half by simmering and add a dollop of alcohol as a preservative. Apply as needed.

Henna has been in recorded use as a coloring agent since before Cleopatra's time. The Egyptians avidly used this dye to obtain a bright auburn tint. The deep color was so favored by the queen's court that henna was used not only to dye the hair, but also the fingernails and the palms of the hands.

While henna has fallen behind the modern dyes, it continues to be used around the world. Since its definite red to flaming orange color sometimes lasts as long as six months, it must be used with caution. A patch test is vital. Because of its intensity of color, and varying conditions of hair, some users have unfortunately been left with strange shades after failing to patch test one small section of their hair before proceeding. The safest arrangement would be to have your hairdresser make the test and apply the henna for you.

Henna does not disturb the molecular structure of the hair as do the chemical dyes. Its application coats the hair shafts, and thus it also increases the body of the hair. Since its effect varies on different hair textures, you must be prepared for a variance from the exact shade you want. Actually, a patch test should be made of any dye before use.

With practice, warm brown tones can be acquired from the henna powder when it is combined with other vegetable dyes. A mixture of one-fourth henna and three-fourths camomile will bring a warm chestnut color to fading brown hair.

A half-and-half combination of henna and camomile will develop a reddish brown tone to the same hair. Again, this can vary with each head of hair, according to its characteristics. Henna applied to white or grey hair will bring about a flaming orange color. Obviously, henna should be avoided by those with this type of coloring.

For a true red color, combine henna powder with boiling water into a thin paste. Brush this paste throughout the hair and then, to insure complete coverage, comb the hair carefully without pulling, over and over.

Arrange a steaming towel, comfortably warm, around the head turban-style. Wear this for thirty minutes while the color develops. Keep the towel moist and warm by wringing it out as needed in hot water and re-covering the head.

After the color has developed, shampoo the scalp and hair well and rinse thoroughly. Remember, pure henna brings a deep, rich red to the hair, without sublety, so be sure this is the color you want before you begin.

In addition to working on problem hair by correcting the diet to supply the needed nutrients for good hair growth, you might want to try one of the following suggestions from our grandmothers and great grandmothers which has been used to prevent loss of hair.

1. Mix two heaping tablespoons of sea salt into one quart of boiling water and allow it to cool before using. Rub a small amount through the scalp daily, continuing to shampoo as needed.

2. Fill a small jar with powdered lobelia. Mix brandy and sweet almond oil in equal parts and add as much of the mixture as the powdered lobelia will absorb. Mix well and allow the compound to stand three or four days. Apply to the roots of the hair by rubbing in daily with the fingertips.

3. Cut a small onion in half and rub the scalp with it just before retiring. The onion juice is supposed to stimulate the skin and invigorate the roots of the hair. Pin a cloth around the hair or wear a curler bonnet. Shampoo with soft water and castile or herbal shampoo in the morning and use a last rinse of apple cider vinegar in the water.

4. Simmer four large handfuls of leaves from the box plant in a covered saucepan for twenty minutes. Allow the brew to steep overnight before straining and adding any desired scent. Use daily as a scalp wash.

5. This recipe is supposed not only to prevent loss of hair, but also to keep it from turning grey. Mix one pint of bay rum and one or two ounces, depending upon the amount of natural oil in the hair, of neat's-foot oil. Blend together thoroughly and apply with the fingertips to the scalp, rubbing into the roots of the hair every night.

CHAPTER ELEVEN

Hand Care and Cures

Good hand care should begin early in life. If every woman knew that the condition of her hands in her mature years would either confirm or deny a youthful appearance, she would give as much attention to her hands as to her face. For the smoothest complexion and the trimmest body will not disguise coarse, reddened or rough hands.

Uneven nails, hangnails and stunted nail growth all mar a woman's beauty. Continued abuse by exposure to harsh weather, dirt, grime, water, detergents and other chemicals can make a soft, well-shaped hand unattractive. Even an occupation as enjoyable as gardening without gloves coarsens the hands.

It is common to see chafed, work-roughened hands on many young women today. By the time these women have reached middle age, their hands will be almost completely ruined if their care consists solely of the hit-or-miss use of some ineffective lotion once or twice a day.

Summer hand care is just as important as wintertime care. Long hours in the swimming pool, the ocean, or exposure to excessive sun rays can dry the skin until it resembles parchment. For this kind of damage, creams rubbed into the skin are seldom sufficient for repair. The moisture itself has been removed from the tissue and only with its restoration can the skin again become soft and elastic.

Restoring moisture to damaged, dried skin is not an easy matter. But by avoiding harmful habits, massaging frequently with various herbal, fruit and vegetable juices, ending with a covering of a nourishing skin cream, trouble can be prevented and improvement gained.

The rigors of winter weather can sap the moisture and oils from unprotected hands. Constant care should be given during the cold months. Gloves should always be worn, creams applied as a protective coating against harsh weather, and cosmetic gloves worn at night when they are needed. In fact, these night gloves should become a part of your beauty wardrobe.

Housework probably takes the greatest toll of hands, but it need not do so. With a careful analysis of one's duties, chores or obligations, a program can be mapped out that will insure hand protection during every chore, as well as follow-up care afterwards. Of course, rubber gloves should always be worn when the hands are immersed in any cleaning solution.

For those who have easily roughened skin, even daily hand washing and bathing can pose a problem if one uses an alkaline soap. Those soaps strip away the natural acid mantle native to healthy skin and leave it vulnerable to easy attack and penetration.

Many women have found that after washing the hands, a simple rinsing in a mild vinegar-water solution will eliminate skin drying, chapping and other irritations. We remind you that all soaps should be of an acid nature for skin protection. These soaps are usually made of vegetable and/or herbal matter. They are cleansing while they help to maintain moisture.

An interesting formula of several generations ago, for those who wanted to avoid any and all soaps, is an old French recipe for a product which used to be sold commercially all over France. Because one of the required ingredients in Amandine is vague in description, and probably is not obtainable on today's market, you might want to pass this one up and go on to the next formula which not only is successful in preparation, but is also delightful to use.

But just in case you locate the missing neutral almond shaving cream or come across an old-time pharmacist or barber who can help you, here it is.

AMANDINE

3 ounces honey
1 ounce powdered gum arabic
1½ ounces neutral almond shaving cream
1 pound cold-pressed sweet almond oil
½ teaspoon perfumed oil

Rub the gum arabic and honey into a thick paste. This is a slow, arduous procedure and requires a strong arm. Add the shaving cream and beat until the mixture becomes homogenized. Pour the almond oil in a slow, thin stream into the mixture, beating constantly. If the oil flows too fast, the mixture does not blend, and the Amandine becomes oily instead of jelly-like and transparent as it will if properly prepared. After the transparent stage has been reached, beat in the perfumed oil.

At one time it was easy enough to purchase the prepared Amandine compound, even in this country. But along with pure rose water and other simple but delightful preparations, it was displaced by modern concoctions that are not as effective as natural products. These items are obtainable only from shops specializing in old-fashioned items, though some pharmacies still carry a few natural preparations.

HONEY CREAM FOR THE HANDS

¼ ounce white wax
¼ ounce spermaceti
½ ounce sweet almond oil
4 ounces honey
Few drops perfumed oil or perfume

Dissolve the wax and spermaceti over hot water. Stir in the almond oil and honey. Blend well and when nearly cool, beat in the perfume. Pour into wide-mouthed cosmetic jars.

For cleansing without soap, dip into the paste and rub it thoroughly into the hands under running water. The water must be warm enough to make the paste easily spreadable. While the hands are still warm, rub them briskly with toweling.

Women of long ago cherished the appearance of pretty hands probably more than many do today. They devised every possible trick for retaining a soft skin. It was in much earlier times that recipes for cosmetic gloves were formulated. And this all-night treatment is worth the slight annoyance of going to bed with gloves on.

Certainly, in our busy world of today there is not time to wander around all day with cream-lathered hands covered with gloves, while waiting for the softening process to take place. Now more than ever, since we so value "getting twenty-four hours out of every day," sleeping with cosmetic gloves on is a very practical thing to do. And what a joy to awaken in the morning with attractive hands, developed while we were asleep.

There are many favored recipes for this preparation, and after experimenting a bit, you can create your own, tailoring it specifically to your personal requirements.

COSMETIC GLOVES

2 egg yolks
2 tablespoons oil of sweet almond
1 teaspoon tincture of benzoin
1 tablespoon rose water
1 pair old white kid gloves, 2 sizes larger than your regular size

Beat the egg yolks until they are bright yellow. Whip in the almond oil and mix well. Add the benzoin, drop by drop, beating all the while. Blend in the rose water.

Lining the gloves with a coating of this healing and beautifying mixture is the next step. There are several approaches. You might turn the gloves inside out and paint every area well with the mixture, then carefully turn them right side out again. Perhaps spreading the mixture into the gloves with a flat wooden tongue depressor or an old emery board is the easiest method.

Kid gloves are preferable to cotton gloves, because of the tendency of cotton to absorb the paste. Hands more easily absorb the rich oils and liquids when encased in kid. And there is less chance of soiling the bed linens. But be sure the gloves are large enough to contain the paste and your hands.

Chapped hands offer a challenge, because usually the habit of acquiring them must first be broken. Many times, simple habitual carelessness causes chapping. Few people take the time to dry their hands completely. This one correction alone can sometimes eliminate the problem.

A mixture of quince seed and whiskey heals and smoothes chapped hands. The recipe permits a choice of consistency. For a thin lotion, use fewer seeds; for thicker, more seeds.

Put the seeds into a jar and add enough whiskey to cover them. This will thicken as the seeds dissolve, at which time you add more whiskey until you have the consistency you desire.

There are several other good recipes for helping hands that never seem to heal, but continue from one chapped or roughened state to another. Choose one or more of the following formulas and decide on the mixture that brings you the best results.

OLIVE-CAMPHOR BALLS

½ ounce spermaceti
½ ounce white wax

¼ ounce finely powdered camphor
olive oil

Mix the spermaceti, wax and camphor together after melting and bind with enough olive oil to create a very stiff paste. Roll this mixture into balls and use after washing the hands or immersing them in water.

ALMOND BALLS FOR CHAPPED HANDS

1 ounce spermaceti
3 tablespoons sweet almond oil

1 teaspoon honey
1 ounce powdered camphor

Melt the spermaceti and beat in the almond oil, honey and camphor. Pack into a small box to create a bar when cold, or roll into balls between the palms of the hands.

CREAM FOR CHAPPED SKIN

½ ounce white wax
6 tablespoons sweet almond oil

2 ounces rose water
1 teaspoon cod liver oil

Melt the wax with the oils and then very slowly, beat in the rose water. It is necessary to add the rose water drop by drop, beating all the while with a fork in order to blend it with the other ingredients. Pour into jars and use daily.

Another nourishing hand protector aids in keeping skin smooth and unwrinkled when used frequently enough.

COCOA CREAM CERATE

1 ounce cocoa butter
1 ounce white wax

4 tablespoons sesame seed oil

Melt all the ingredients together and use before retiring. This is also a good cream to apply before doing heavy housework.

Once hand discolorations have begun, it is no easy matter to remove them. Some vegetables and fruits will act as a bleach on the hands with the same success as on the face, if the stains are not too deeply embedded. But others, if long neglected, will need a more heroic effort. The following recipe is for the hands only and must not be used to the point of irritation.

ALMOND MEAL FOR REMOVING DISCOLORATION ON THE HANDS

8 ounces fine almond powder
1 ounce curd soap, powdered
1 ounce castile soap, powdered

¾ ounce orris root, powdered
2 ounces cuttlefish bone, powdered

Mix all the ingredients together and sift through a fine sieve. Wet the hands and dip into a container of this meal and rub together before rinsing and applying a hand cream.

CHAPTER TWELVE

Bathing for Body and Soul

Bathing has long been recognized as a vital part of any beauty regimen. Cleopatra's sixty-nine baths a day in ass's milk were perhaps the height of this pursuit for charm. But while she may have been a raving beauty with skin like velvet, this indulgence seems ludicrous to us now.

The effects she sought are far more easily achieved today without an entourage of animals and their keepers. To enjoy the same results that Cleopatra sought, try pouring a cup of powdered skim milk into a tub of warm water and swishing it about until it dissolves. This is used by many women today as a means of producing a smooth-textured, satiny skin. Towel yourself dry after such a bath without additional rinsing, and you're a modern Cleopatra.

Beauty bathing should always be a pleasant occupation, something to be anticipated and easily taken. There is just as much to be gained from a relaxing, soothing, beautifying bath as any other approach to body loveliness.

The early Greeks took daily baths to refresh themselves and to increase their vigor. The height of luxury ablutions en masse probably took place in Rome. The evidence of their appreciation of leisurely bathing can be seen in the ruins of their once magnificent establishments. Wherever they lived, there are remnants of these huge centers.

Tiled and marbled bath ruins in Pompeii are as grand as their local city hall. Hot and cold ducts brought water of the desired temperature to varying sizes of marble pools. After a long soaking, a bather selected his scented oil or perfume with which he lathered himself.

In one Roman establishment of nearly two thousand years ago, a bather was able to choose from over two dozen different baths—hot, cold, fruit, vegetable, milk, honey and so on. But the oil bath was the most popular, just as it is today.

The oil bath has many uses. Helpless to do otherwise, we daily subject our bodies to the ravaging effects of detergents, chemicals, dyes from clothing, smoke, gasoline fumes and sprays. Sun worshippers add the drying qualities of extensive sunbathing to this. Harsh winds and exposure compound the damage.

The oil bath becomes a necessity today, after all this devastating exposure and irritation. Also, bathing in a solution of oil and water helps to restore some of the moisture we tend to lose as we grow older.

There is great pleasure and benefit to be had from a bath laced with oil that is so reviving to a heat- or winter-dried body. The pores actually seem to be renewed by this soothing treatment. The oil clings to the skin, and even after a brisk towelling it penetrates and creates a lithe, supple feeling.

Though there are multitudes of bathing preparations on the market, it is easy enough to prepare your own. In this way you can avoid the products containing mineral oil, a by-product of crude oil and of no value to the skin, though it is frequently used in commercial bath oil preparations.

By bathing daily we are not only freshening our bodies and removing normal and natural waste accumulations. We are also removing the external collection of toxins from sprays, fallout and other sources that coat our sensitive skins.

Though bathing should be a serious undertaking with enough friction applied to cleanse the pores, it should also be a relaxing and enjoyable experience. In the tub one can shed tensions and worries. The easing of ligaments and muscles tends to release a tight brow and remove frown lines that can become habitual. Rest and bathing can be successfully combined to produce a state of tranquillity that rest alone cannot give us.

Convenience should dictate bathtime, but once the time is decided upon, the bath should become routine. Early morning baths can be an introduction to a rewarding day. This gentle easing into one's schedule can make the difference between pleasure in one's work and a reluctant acknowledgment of duties. On the other hand, an evening bath can soothe away the difficulties of the day and help prepare the way to a full night's restful sleep.

Bath water should never be extreme in temperature. The practice of yoga, on which many sensible health rules are based, suggests that the body must never be shocked. Don't suddenly plunge into a brisk shower or hot or cold tub. The shock to the body is brutal and should be avoided. One should also avoid the highly touted hot shower with a sudden change to cold. The violent reaction of the nervous system to such treatment cannot be considered beneficial.

Fill a tub with comfortably warm water. Have everything at hand that you will need, in order to avoid any interruptions. Experiment with bathing solutions; change about and vary your bath while you discover a new experience.

For those who enjoy a smooth, silky body and who want to experiment with homemade oils, mix one cup of corn, safflower or other nut or vegetable oil with one tablespoon of herbal shampoo. If you prefer a scented bath oil, add several drops of perfume or toilet water to the mixture. Or you might add oil of rose geranium, lemon verbena or other scented oil.

Place this mixture in a blender and beat at a high speed to emulsify the solution. Or use an egg beater and beat until well blended. Bottle and use four tablespoons to a bath. Pour the solution directly under the water faucet so the force of the falling water will blend the bath oil with the water.

From southern England comes the recipe for a bath that is beautiful in thought and performance. North of Stonehenge, a meadow is thickly carpeted with the golden camomile flower. An elderly villager spoke to me of the benefits she had enjoyed all her life from the lovely plants. As a young girl she had gathered the flowers to prepare a rinse for her hair. It added, she said, touches of gold to dull blonde or mousy tones.

As she grew older, she gathered a basket of camomile flowers and dropped them into her bath. They soothed as nothing else could, she said. Later in life, she learned to brew tisanes, or herbal teas, from the healing and beautifying plant to allay a nervousness that afflicted her. Whether from her brew, her bath or both, or from her knowledge that nature heals by offering her plants to be used in a multitude of ways, this composed woman lived happily in her village, never a stone's throw away from her beloved camomile meadows.

For a bath of camomile, brew a double handful of the flower heads into a strong infusion, steep for fifteen or twenty minutes and strain and pour into the bath water.

For other pretty and soothing baths, fill a large glass jar with the dried petals of scented herbs and flowers, either separately or combined. You can use lemon verbena (our grandmothers scented linens with it), lavender, rose geranium, marjoram, nasturtiums, rose petals or bergamot.

When you are ready for your scented tub, steep a cupful of the mixed petals and leaves in a pint of boiling water for fifteen minutes or so. Strain the liquid into your filled tub.

Wild herbs are plentiful and easy to come by if you are adventuresome. Dandelion leaves, stinging nettle, (Be careful! Handle with gloves.) blackberry and raspberry leaves, when thoroughly dried and crumbled into a large bowl with scalding water poured over them, make an excellent addition to the bath.

After steeping the leaves for twenty minutes, strain the liquid into your bath water. For the best results it is necessary to bathe in this solution three or four times a week, with a fresh solution used each time. An excellent bath for strengthening the body, it is cleansing and relaxing at the same time.

A bath that supposedly kept Ninon de Lenclos, the famous French beauty, well preserved into her eighties was a simple mixture that sounds incredibly easy. For this internationally acclaimed bath, mix a cup each of dried lavender flowers, mint leaves, rosemary, comfrey roots and thyme. Place all in a cloth bag, or catch up in a cotton square and tie the ends together. Pour boiling water over the mixture and steep for fifteen minutes. Put the entire mixture, bag and all, into the tub and fill with water.

Pine needles, balsam, sage or other pungent scents all contribute to a wondrous bath. Their resinous qualities heal an irritated skin. These, too, should be steeped in hot water first, to bring out their oils or scents. Although one of these baths taken occasionally can be pleasant, for more definite results they should be used over a period of two months or so with some regularity.

A cup or two of bran, tied into a cheesecloth or muslin bag and swished about in the water, is a helpful addition to the bath. The bran contains oils and vegetable hormones and imparts smoothness to the entire body. You can also use the bran bag as a washcloth and give a fine luster to the skin.

There is another recipe using bran to soften hard, resistant skin and refine body pores. Mix equal parts of powdered bran (use the blender) and oatmeal. To one pint of the mixture, add one-half cup of grated vegetable soap and one ounce of powdered orris root (optional). Fill small bags to use as washcloths in the tub.

That same oatmeal we have admired as food, masque or lotion, is an old favorite in the bath and has found its devotees around the world. To avoid clogging the bath drain, put the oatmeal in a cloth bag, swish it around in the tub and rub directly on the skin after both are wet. Or you can reduce the oatmeal to the finest powder in the blender—or buy oatmeal flour—and add a cup to the tub of warm water. Always use old-fashioned oatmeal rather than the instant kind.

A salt bag kept near the tub to rub on your skin insures a finely textured skin surface by removing hardened layers of dead tissue. Fill a small bag with sea salt, just enough to be handled easily. No soap is needed when you use this invigorating scrubber. And the minerals in the salt will benefit your skin.

Also, keep a bowl of sea salt in the bathroom. Even during a shower, after wetting your body, you can rub yourself all over with handfuls of the salt before stepping back under the spray for a rinse-off. Roughened areas will become silky in texture very quickly.

Many countries have contributed to the infinite variety of baths that make bathing more meaningful than merely getting clean. The sauna bath of the Scandinavian countries cleans the pores, stimulates the skin and invigorates the body. The popularity of the sauna has spread around the world, and one can find such accommodations in almost any city in America now. There are sauna baths for the private home and even do-it-yourself kits for constructing these units in your basement.

Several European countries continue to offer mud baths to which people have made beauty and health pilgrimages for centuries. The minerals found in the black flowing mud in parts of Germany increase the circulation of the blood and add vitality to skin and body. Andorra, the tiny country hidden between France and Spain, offers sulphur baths that seem to take years of fatigue away. France claims that her own mineral baths clear the constitution and restore youth and joie de vivre.

But you can have baths just as exotic as these without leaving your own bathroom. Run a tub of water warm enough to dissolve one pound of Epsom salts. Relax in the tub for fifteen minutes, then rub the entire body with a towel, briskly enough to remove all dead skin. The use of Epsom salts also aids the body in removal of toxins that exit through the skin. But this bath should not be taken too frequently. It is more to be used as a restorative for stiff or overworked muscles and ligaments, besides aiding in toxin removal. The salt water bath is similar. You will feel as if you have just had a swim in the ocean if you dip into your supply of sea salt instead of the usual table salt. Use up to one pound of salt in the tub. It's all according to how much surf you want! This bath is a real treasure for firming sagging, flabby skin.

Apple cider vinegar offers superb results in relieving aching muscles or itching skin. The water takes on a velvety quality after the vinegar is added, and it is softening to the skin. Pour one cup of apple cider vinegar into your tub of warm water. Soak for fifteen or twenty minutes and allow the mixture to soothe both skin and body.

The sponge bath has its place as a survivor from the Victorian age. This abbreviated bath was easier to take than a regular one requiring kettles of water to be heated and poured and, later, emptied from the tub.

One of the world's greatest beauties, Sarah Bernhardt, attributed her own high sense of spirit and life both on the stage and off to her favorite bath which she called an *eau sédative*. At the age of fifty-five the Divine Sarah had the appearance of a woman half her age.

Her recipe calls for two ounces of spirits of ammonia, two ounces of camphor, one cup of sea salt and two cups of ethyl alcohol. Instructions say to place all the ingredients in a quart bottle and fill the bottle with boiling water. Shake vigorously before using. Use the liquid at room temperature.

When using the *eau sédative*, stand in a tub and with a soft cloth dip into a bowl of the liquid. Rub gently all over the body. Afterwards rub dry with a towel. This soothing sponge bath is reputed to remove soreness and fatigue from the body. In addition, according to the celebrated actress, there is an increase in circulation, a sense of relaxation, and a desire to sleep. This solution is to be used only in stress situations.

Grandmother's beauty bath, from the same period, sounds like a sturdy, no-nonsense approach to loveliness. Though it seems complicated, it also sounds edible. And since Grandmother used all the products of nature around her back door and emerged with a beautiful complexion even in her older years, then her favorite bath might be regarded with respect.

For the bath she indulged in probably no more than once weekly, Grandmother used the following recipe:

- 2 pounds of oatmeal
- 2 pounds of bran
- 2 pounds of non-pearled barley
- 2 pounds of brown rice
- 8 ounces of bicarbonate of soda
- 1 pound of dried lavender flowers
- 1 pound of bay leaves

Boil all ingredients together for one hour in a quantity of rainwater. Strain and add two quarts to a tub of water. Reserve the remainder for other baths.

Grandmother's recipes were seldom specific down to the last measurement, and in this one too she has left it up to you as to the quantity of water to use. Since one bath requires two quarts, I should imagine that it was made up in quantities of at least eight quarts.

This would require an enormous container, plus extra refrigerating space for keeping the leftover liquid, so perhaps the recipe should be cut in half. If you are of an experimental nature, then proceed from there, aiming at what you believe would be the right proportions for this old recipe.

It should be remembered that any herbal or beauty bath does not require additional bathing to remove the effects or residue from the skin. Vigorous towelling takes care of that. In this way you retain all possible benefits from these calming, beautifying and nourishing baths.

While beauty baths can consist of a multitude of lotions and brews concocted for addition to the tub, one unusual beauty bath should not be ignored. This is an equally famous bath that requires no water. The dry bath can have beneficial effects on the skin of the body when correctly practiced. The French seem to have devised this intriguing and effective method of dry bathing, though it is practiced in other areas of the world.

The *gant de massage,* or massage glove, could become a weekly practice for those wanting to keep the skin in its finest condition. The purpose of these rough-appearing gloves is to remove the dried and dead skin from the body surface. Used dry, the glove brushes off accumulated dead cells from body pores and permits the skin to breathe. Blood circulation is increased and toxins lying on the surface skin are disposed of more quickly.

The dry bath is best used just before retiring, for it is conducive to sleep. The French declare it is a cure for insomnia. Whether this is true or not, it does refresh and tone the body, even as it relaxes it. In addition, the friction glove, as it is also called cleanses and refines the pores.

This is not accomplished overnight. But when practiced over a substantial period of time, there should be a gradual improvement in the pores. No rough exertions should be used with the friction glove. The heavily textured fabric makes only the lightest movements necessary.

Switch the glove from the left to the right hand in order to reach all parts of the body. Massage gently in an upward sweeping motion. Don't fail to cover the lower part of the derrière, especially for those who are chair-bound in an office. In this area where roughness and even calloused skin are the occupational hazards of constant chair sitting, the friction glove can polish the skin as smooth as the skin on the forearm or face. Heels, elbows and knees also profit from the dry bath treatment. No part of the body should be ignored, but pay careful attention to these trouble spots.

Friction gloves are made from many materials, originally from hemp. This sturdy material resembles an instrument of torture and indeed can be if improperly used. But if it is rubbed over the entire body, one feels brand-new. Other fabrics used for the gloves include heavy cotton, wool, horsehair and, now, plastic. Though the plastic is hygienic and easily kept clean, it does not produce the same effect as the more resilient natural fibers.

A very fine friction glove can be grown at home right in your own garden. Simply plant a crop of the old-fashioned dishcloth gourds. When the crop ripens, cut the gourd away from its vine and allow it to dry for several days. Then carefully cut away the outside shell until you expose the web-like interior. Place this skeletal mesh to dry in the sunshine for a week. When it is completely dried, shake the stiffened web free of the seeds and voilà! You have a *gant de massage* exactly like those sold in Paris bath shops. For a few cents worth of seeds, you can grow a year's supply, and even have enough to give away as presents.

The only place in our country I know of that still carries these old-fashioned seeds in their stock is the George W. Park Company, Greenwood, South Carolina, 29646.

Remember to exercise caution in the use of the friction glove. A weekly dry bath is frequent enough. In all matters of health and personal body care, be practical when you choose that which appeals either to your sense of adventure, luxury, timeliness or need.

Experiment with caution; consider your skin texture, the delicacy of your tissue, your allergic reactions if any and the general physical condition of your body. A rule one learns in the practice of yoga is that no two bodies are alike; therefore, you must never compare yourself to another, but answer the personal needs of your own body.

If the dry bath feels too severe for you, try using the friction glove in your regular bath. Soap and water soften its action, and this technique is a beneficial method of cleansing your body.

CHAPTER THIRTEEN

Beauty foods

We should cherish the velvety-textured skin we are born with as early in life as we learn to care for any other part of the body. We do not consider it unusual to come into the world with a perfect complexion and to have it for most of our early days. But as we get older, we accept a poor skin condition as our natural lot. Other than dabbing on an occasional cream or using concealing makeup, we often do little to fight the change from living, vibrant tissue to tired, patchy skin with many troubles.

As said earlier, the first approach to maintaining a good skin condition is to eat properly. Dependent upon nutritional supply and internal well-being, the skin will be healthy, performing its tasks and presenting a softly elastic condition or it will be malfunctioning, with unsightly blemishes due to noxious wastes.

Lack of proper nutrition paints a picture of age and exhaustion on both face and body, no matter what the numerical years. Defective eating habits can mar the most attractive face and figure, while a diet that contains all the essentials of good health will bring color to withered cheeks, sparkle to dulled eyes and tone to a dreary appearance.

Part of the cause of today's poor nutrition lies in our stereotyped notions of good meals. It seems to us that a breakfast of juice, bacon and eggs or cold cereal, toast and beverage offers a splendid source of energy for our working day. Undoubtedly, this was true, once. But these days, while stuffing ourselves with calories, we really starve on such a meal.

For this breakfast is not what it seems. The juice is frozen, canned or synthetic; the bacon probably chemically cured; the eggs, if not cold-storage, are at least non-fertilized, and the toast is made from white bread completely stripped of any real food value. The cold cereal has been popped, sugar-coated, roasted or otherwise tortured and changed from its natural grain.

Devitalized foods in the diet will be improperly digested and play havoc with the internal system, breeding countless ills and destroying beauty. Among these useless and damaging foods are all white flour products, polished rice, refined sugar and anything that has been canned, processed, added to, taken from, heated or preserved.

Instead of these foods, we should seek out whole grain flours and cereals, unprocessed meats, raw honey or raw sugar and fresh fruits, and vegetables, organic if possible. The foods sold in the market today are producing a country full of wan young people, destined to early aging and illness. The trend of producing non-food products seems to be expanding around the world. Various reasons are given for this: the population is too large to provide with organic foods which are too expensive to produce, a general scarcity of food, the ease of transporting and storing processed foods and so on.

Some countries are refusing to follow this trend, but all too often one can see concessions made to the times as the small grocery gives way to the supermarket in which food comes from huge warehouses or refining machinery instead of nearby sources.

The sheer joy of marketing in an area where the fruits and vegetables glisten with moisture that came from the fields that very morning, rather than from the supermarket sprinkling can, cannot be duplicated.

Natural foods will bring you natural beauty. A diet that concentrates on raw, fresh foods will help to dispose of an oily complexion, enlarged pores and many other skin problems. Soft, nutritionless foods will lead to early wrinkles, sagging muscles and fatigue. It was Helena Rubinstein who said that health is the well from which a woman can draw perpetual youth.

When we care for our hair, nurture our skin and exercise our bodies, we are attempting to hold on to the qualities associated with youth. If everyone would treat his body as a growing plant, needing constant attention, and supply it with all the nutrients required for growth and maintenance, one's body at seventy could be as well formed, the hair as lustrous and the step as quick and positive as it was fifty years earlier.

We are too quick to accept with defeat those depressing symptoms of age, and consider them to be normal and natural. Vitality will come to any body if it is properly fed and cared for. You cannot cut off the source of invaluable vitamins and minerals from your body and not expect to pay for it. Today's empty foods are producing tired women, old before their time, and have driven them to the use of an excess of artificial makeup.

A quick way to ruin, particularly facial ruin, is through fad diets. No matter how desperate, one should not succumb to these incredible diets which eliminate all vegetables or all meat or all grains to concentrate on one item and "watch the pounds melt away."

The pounds may disappear, briefly, but so does one's stamina, the life in the skin and hair and one's resistance to infection. Starvation diets are just that. They have no value beyond a crash plan to lose a few pounds which will quickly return as soon as the usual food pattern is resumed, leaving hidden inner damage behind.

It is much wiser and easier than becoming involved with a fad diet to revise one's food plan according to natural health rules. The weight problem then takes care of itself. And by learning to use natural organic food as much as possible and eliminating all non-foods, you can expect a blemish-free complexion and a youthful body. Younger women will be able to extend their beauty well into their older years without the usual middle-age problems.

One idea of good nutrition is based on the system of diet given in the magazine *Prevention.* Instead of eating meat every day as is the custom in our country, better results can be expected from using meat only two or three times a week. There are other excellent sources of protein as well.

Vegetables should be organic to be nutritious, grown without chemical fertilizers, without sprays and not frozen, canned or wilted. If you cannot always get organic vegetables, there are ways to improvise. One of these is to grow your own vegetables, right in your kitchen, with no more than a seed-sprouter and a bag of seeds. This method produces a delicious array of fresh, green, vitamin-rich "vegetables," which will provide you with a crop of greens with less trouble than it takes to pinch the turnips in the supermarket to find the least shrivelled.

You can grow sprouts from lentils, mung beans, soy, millet, alfalfa, barley and other grains, nuts and seeds. All produce a quick crop that will provide fresh vitamin-packed salad material or food to be quickly steamed.

These kitchen-grown crops are small, of course, but extremely concentrated in food value, and careful planning can produce enough in the tiniest of kitchens to provide adequately for the day's needs, even for a fairly large family.

The bean sprouter you can buy at the health food store comes with directions; you can also easily grow sprouts in an ordinary jar. Put enough seeds in the bottom of a pint canning jar to fill one-sixth of the jar. Cover with water and allow seeds to soak for eighteen to twenty-four hours. Pour off the water (it is very nutritious—use in soup) and rinse the seeds. Cover the jar with a piece of cheesecloth or nylon mesh held down with a rubber band. Night and morning rinse the seeds several times by pouring the water in and out through the cheesecloth or mesh. No water must be left in the jar, but the seeds should be thoroughly washed. The seeds sprout and are ready to eat—they grow to a couple of inches—by the end of three days ordinarily, although seeds differ in the length of time they need to sprout.

Raw vegetables, green salads and whole grain foods all contribute to the internal cleanliness which creates external beauty. Instead of consuming starchy, useless foods that lie dormant and cause putrefaction, rely on the enzyme-rich fresh food to keep the body beautiful and clean.

As we've said before, the marvelous composition of the body demands individual attention and treatment. To bring yourself to peak performance and attractiveness, you must scout out your own dietary needs much as a sleuth detects signs and symbols. Then, remaining within the natural foods rules of diet, you can discover the solutions to your particular problems.

If your skin is dry, rough or flaky, concentrate on those foods which bring relief to this problem, and use some of them daily. These are foods rich in vitamin A such as sweet potatoes, carrots, turnip greens, parsley, raw spinach, pimentoes, dandelion greens, chard, fish liver and vegetable oils, eggs and dairy products.

Normal skin functions will be determined to a great degree by sufficient intake and assimilation of the B vitamins. Fatigue and nervousness, which manifests itself in blotchy, lifeless or pimply skin, can result from a vitamin B deficiency. Since the entire B-complex family of vitamins is responsible for everything from an energy source to faulty digestion leading to constipation, you can see the necessity of getting sufficient daily quantities of this beauty vitamin. For no skin can remain clear and glowing when the internal system is clogged, and no body can be pushed beyond exhaustion and not appear ravaged with poor health.

In addition to its role as a cold inhibitor, vitamin C is being revealed as a bastion against aging. It is small wonder that there has been a run on the market, and sources of vitamin C in supplement form are sometimes difficult to find.

But one can always obtain this incredible and youthifying vitamin from fresh fruits and vegetables.

Creating firmness in tissue and resistance to other aging factors, vitamin C taken daily becomes as much a need as the nightly creaming of the face.

Lowered resistance to infections comes from a lack of vitamins A and C. This means that any skin infection can assume larger proportions because of the body's inability to overcome attacks made upon it.

Being soluble, vitamin C mixes readily with body fluids and thus can easily be lost whenever the body disposes of liquids through normal processes. Also much of its value is lost in cooking and careless handling of foods.

Squeezing the juice from citrus fruits and throwing away the fruit itself is an extravagant waste of vitamin C. In addition to this loss, there is also the loss of the invaluable vitamin P which abounds in the white membranous coating of the inner citrus peels. As mentioned in Chapter Seven, the combination of vitamins C and P plus rutin are excellent means of correcting the small broken veins that can mar an otherwise attractive face.

City-bound people are usually woefully short on the beauty vitamin D. Perhaps this is why these urbanites rush to the seashores and lakes each summer in order to compensate for the lack of this vitamin that comes from the sun's rays. Though moderate amounts of sunshine will amply supply the body's needs for vitamin D, unfortunately many health seekers overexpose themselves to the sun's rays and do as much harm as good.

It is far better to depend on moderate exposure to the sun and rely on fish liver oils for good measure in getting one's quota of vitamin D. This vitamin is only infrequently found in our regular foods. Raw milk in the summer when the cows have eaten green pasturage is quite high in vitamin D. Egg yolk also has vitamin D.

Since this beauty vitamin is a co-factor in calcium assimilation, its deficiency shows itself in the restlessness and nervousness indicative of mal-absorption of calcium.

Skin can be healthy and vibrant, but faulty functioning due to a missing vitamin or sketchy area in the diet, can begin to produce signs of premature age. There is no positive answer as to the exact cause of the unsightly brown spots that appear when one is in one's forties, but there have been many suggestions.

Called liver spots, or age signs, these persistent spots will sometimes respond to a corrected intake of vitamin E and massages of the vitamin which is then left on the skin overnight. These unsightly discolorations obviously require many years of deficient or faulty nutrition in order to appear. In consequence, you must be patient as you await results and not be discouraged after only a few applications. Many months are sometimes necessary to aid in the toning down or complete removal of the spots that spell old age to many women.

Since foods for beauty and health include so many raw fruits and vegetables, we have listed numerous salads below. If just one meal a day is built around such a salad, you will be working actively toward a rejuvenated body and glowing face.

ZUCCHINI SALAD

½ cup raw sliced zucchini
½ cup green pepper strips
4 sliced raw mushrooms

SPINACH SALAD

¼ pound raw spinach
¼ cup chopped parsley
½ chopped onion
1 grated carrot
1 clove garlic

WATERCRESS AND AVOCADO SALAD

1 cup watercress
½ large avocado, or 1 small one
4 sliced radishes
½ cup raw green peas

CABBAGE AND CARROT SALAD

1 cup finely grated green cabbage
1 carrot, grated
1 apple, chopped

CAULIFLOWER SALAD

1 cup sliced raw cauliflower
¼ cup chopped parsley
½ cup chopped celery
1 small cucumber, sliced
1 small green pepper, chopped

SPROUT SALAD

1 cup any bean, nut, or seed sprouts
2 tomatoes
1 cup endive
1 small cucumber

SPROUT AND EGG SALAD

1 cup any type sprouts
1 hardboiled egg, chopped
½ cup chopped celery
½ grated carrot

TURNIP SALAD

1 small turnip, grated
1 carrot, grated
½ cup celery, chopped
Romaine or other lettuce leaves

CHICKORY AND DANDELION SALAD

1 cup chickory greens
1 cup tender spring dandelions
½ cup sliced mushrooms
1 tomato, chopped
1 green pepper, sliced

RADISH-CUCUMBER SALAD

½ cup radishes, sliced thin, with ¼ cup radish leaves, minced
1 cucumber, sliced
1 tomato, sliced
1 onion, chopped

TOMATOES STUFFED WITH SPROUTS

1 tomato shell with insides removed and chopped
½ cup mung sprouts
½ small onion, chopped

GREEN PEA AND MUSHROOM SALAD

1 cup raw green peas
½ cup sliced raw mushrooms
1 cup lettuce, shredded

ASPARAGUS SALAD

1 cup tender parts of raw, green asparagus
1 cup raw cauliflower, sliced
½ cup raw mushrooms, sliced

AVOCADO AND BANANA SALAD

1 small or ½ large avocado, diced
1 banana, sliced
½ cup fresh pineapple, cubed
lettuce leaves
homemade mayonnaise

WALNUT AND NASTURTIUM SALAD

½ cup shelled walnuts
½ dozen nasturtium leaves
several torn lettuce leaves
segments of 1 orange

MANGO AND WATERCRESS SALAD

½ large mango, sliced
1 cup watercress, chopped
¼ cup raw, sliced almonds

PINEAPPLE AND GRAPE SALAD

1 cup fresh pineapple, cubed
1 cup sliced black grapes
½ cup shredded green cabbage
homemade mayonnaise

A simple and good salad dressing for the salads is a vinaigrette sauce, using one tablespoon of apple cider vinegar or lemon juice to three tablespoons of salad oil. Season the vinegar before adding the oil and shake vigorously. You may vary the taste of the dressing by adding grated cheese, minced onion, garlic, sea kelp or any herbal plant, either fresh or dried.

CHAPTER FOURTEEN

Cleanliness From Within

Any machine or device which receives material to produce energy must have its channels of waste disposal kept open and active. Otherwise, trouble develops, and the machine will no longer function adequately.

It sometimes helps to compare the human body with a machine. We can understand the simple logic of a clogged valve or pipe jamming up the works and preventing an efficient operation. And we usually try to keep our machines trouble-free in order to have them function smoothly. But we are often less willing to supervise our body's intake and its waste disposal.

And yet, neglect of the disposal system of the body can lead to damaging physical conditions that become more serious as the indifference persists. Any bit of waste that does not go the usual orderly way will rush to another exit.

The four channels of elimination include the intestines, the kidneys, the lungs and the skin. All wastes from the healthy body will be thrown out through one of these organs and pose no further problem. If the intestines are blocked, flaccid or otherwise malfunctioning, the waste that was intended for the bowel will find its way into another organ of disposal.

Where intestinal elimination is faulty, some of the internal toxins will force their way out of the body through the skin. While this is a safety measure performed by the bloodstream to excrete poisons out of the body and so prevent a more serious internal disturbance, the external skin results can become quite disturbing.

Pimples, blotched, muddy skin tones and sebaceous eruptions can all come from an improperly functioning disposal system in any of the four channels of elimination.

Outer beauty simply and surely depends on inner cleanliness. Creams and lotions become only a palliative treatment of skin ailments until the inner difficulties are met.

That same good nutrition which provides beauty is a prime requisite in correcting faulty body functions. Half of the battle can be won by adjusting the diet to meet all the requirements of good nutrition.

Adequate amounts of liquids are necessary in order to clear the body of toxins. The kidneys play an important role in the eliminative process, and thus in keeping the complexion clear. Approximately twenty gallons of liquid are filtered through the kidneys each day. No more than two quarts of this fluid are excreted while the remainder is recirculated through the body. Water flushing is needed, then, to assist the kidneys in ridding themselves of the concentrated poison which has been strained from the mainstream of the body fluid.

If the wastes are not sufficiently flushed out, the concentration of poisons can create disturbances both inside and outside the body. But the water drinking habit usually has to be cultivated if one is subject to dehydration.

The use of yogurt, the beverage made from kefir grains (similar to buttermilk) and whey helps to encourage good elimination. Yogurt is used in many parts of the world as a mainstay in the diet. And in these areas one finds the sturdiest people, usually free of degenerative diseases and with blemish-free complexions. What is in these foods that have such value in removing wastes from the body?

First and foremost, yogurt and kefir grains supply valuable acids needed for proper digestion of foods. Without this breakdown action, food is not digested and becomes not only unassimilable, but an added burden to the disposal system.

When the friendly bacteria which these products promote in the intestines are in abundance, digestion is improved and elimination normalized.

Both fresh and stewed fruits help keep the eliminative organs working well. An apple a day, peeling and all if it is free of insecticide sprays and wax, aids the absorption of toxins in the digestive tract.

Because of the importance of the kidneys and intestines as organs of disposal, we are inclined to forget that the skin and lungs carry an equally heavy burden. The lungs, in supplying fresh quantities of oxygen, must also remove gaseous impurities. One can deep-breathe to increase the oxygen supply so necessary to a well-functioning body. Shallow breathing limits the oxygen intake as well as exhalation of poisons.

It is just as easy to develop a polluted body through insufficient breathing and exhalation as it is through poor diet. One's health and beauty depend on good breathing habits along with a good diet.

The skin pores must be kept open in order to avoid the blockage that results in infections. Daily cleansing with a complexion brush, occasional facial steaming and exercise will make the blood circulate better, and the natural pore-cleansing will be made easier.

The dry salt-rub and the salt-water bath, as we said in Chapter Twelve, not only make the skin satiny, but also clean away dead cellular wastes very effectively.

Regular exercise should also play a vital part in your plan for correcting elimination. Planned body movement stimulates the sluggish system. Walking, for those who do not care for regular exercises, is one of the finest body toners. All parts of the body, including the organs, receive a gentle massage when one walks. Deep breathing should be combined with walking in order to cleanse the body's airways, force fresh oxygen into all parts of the body and help to expel impurities.

CHAPTER FIFTEEN

Exercises for A Perfect Figure

A compact, firm body that moves with ease, agility and the joy of living is not the exclusive property of youth. One can be lithe and beautiful all one's life with proper care. But unless we do sufficiently exercise all parts of the body, deterioration gains a foothold and the aging process becomes established.

What comes as a gift, and is therefore taken for granted during youth, we must work for during our later years. If planned body movement is begun early enough and is continued throughout life, we can keep at bay the limitations imposed by time.

The reawakening of the body is a most rewarding experience. The most dissolute and neglected figure can be restored to some measure of grace with daily exercises. The overblown bodies one sees everywhere today are prisons that hold beneath excess flesh marvelous structures of physical form.

The body is a wonderful creation. It is only through lack of discipline and knowledge that we lose its original beauty. In yoga practices, the body is considered to be a temple of the living spirit. If this is true, then such a special place should not be abused by demeaning it with folds of flesh or posture that reveals defeat and boredom.

Since it is the highest living creation, the body should live up to its ideal of health and beauty. A planned exercising program will help achieve this goal. If such a program is followed, expansive hips melt away, fleshy, undulating arms become firm, waistlines lose inches, and large thighs diminish. Even the calves of the legs can be whittled down. The poor posture caused by weak, unused muscles and habitual fatigue is replaced by a taller stature and natural ease.

In addition to improving the overall physical condition, daily exercise increases mental vitality. Also, fresh supplies of oxygen and the stimulation of the bloodstream positively affect the complexion.

A determined rather than a frantic approach is the best way to begin. At first, exercise is somewhat like a shot in the arm. One notices an immediate uplift and continues the program with enthusiasm. But caution is needed to temper the over-enthusiastic. Many performers burn themselves out early in their program and become exercise dropouts.

A planned exercise program fitted to your own needs and schedule is easier to stick with after the first novelty has worn away.

Try for balance in your daily exercises. Do not concentrate only on one part of the anatomy. There will be greater dividends if you work for stimulation of the different areas of the whole body.

Deep breathing should accompany exercising in order to supply adequate amounts of oxygen. We can call these deep breaths "beauty breathing," for benefits to every area of the body will increase many times as breathing is coordinated with the physical movements. The end result will be a sparkling complexion and shining eyes as well as a feeling of inner glow.

To practice beauty breathing, lie flat on the floor face up and hold your arms comfortably at your sides. Relax the entire body. Without moving the chest area, slowly inhale through the nostrils with the mouth closed. Try to push the oxygen slowly without lifting the chest, to the lower part of the abdomen. Your abdomen will automatically expand with the increased oxygen supply.

Think of your body as a water pitcher being filled with water from the bottom up. The oxygen will then fill every part of the lungs. Very slowly exhale until the abdomen is flat again.

After practicing this lying down, you should be ready to incorporate it into your other exercises. Beauty breathing may require practice for some days before it is mastered, for it is very different from conventional deep breathing exercises.

Don't overdo it in the beginning. Long accustomed to a sparse oxygen supply and suddenly given an increased amount, you may get dizzy. Beauty breathing should not replace normal breathing. It should be reserved for exercise periods and moments of stress.

Correct posture can mean the difference between an attractive and a nondescript appearance. Walking, standing and sitting with the shoulders comfortably erect, one may help overcome numerous unsuspectedly related problems.

Beautiful carriage develops more elastic muscles in the shoulder area. The downward pull of slumped shoulders not only ages the body both in appearance and in fact, but this rounded position also prevents an adequate supply of oxygen from reaching the inner organs where it is needed. Rounded shoulders emphasize a defeated and negative attitude as they pull the head downward and curve the neck. In this slumped position, the underchin muscles sag into a double chin from the slack muscles which eventually develop.

Another figure fault which results from poor shoulder posture is sagging breasts. As the shoulders bend downard, they allow the weight of the breasts to sink with them. The pectoral muscles lose tone and with their downfall add to the overall condition of poor body tone.

Posture Exercises

1. The following is an excellent morning exercise as it creates a pattern of good posture for the day. Upon arising, stand by an opened window and take a slow, deep, beauty breath. Clasp your hands behind your back and spread the feet about six inches apart. Slowly bend forward at the waist as you

raise your arms upward behind your back, aiming them as high as they can comfortably reach. Do not strain or force.

In the beginning they may rise only a few inches, according to the condition of your body. Very slowly, return your hands to a lightly clasped position behind the back and bring the head up again.

2. In a kneeling position, sit on the heels and place the hands palms down on the front of the thighs. Take a beauty breath and slowly bring the hands up toward the hips by bringing the elbows close to the body. Keep the back straight as you stretch the shoulders backward and expand the chest. Exhale and relax.

3. Lie face down with the palms flat on the floor on either side of the face. Very slowly raise the upper portion of the body from the waist upward, while lifting the hands, palms frontward and remaining to either side of the face. Keep the toes on the floor. Come down slowly.

Another version of this strengthening exercise: take the same face-down position on the floor with the palms flat on the floor. Taking a beauty breath, lift the upper torso and hands simultaneously. Slowly swing the arms back of the body, clasp them and lift them upward. Keep the toes on the floor. Relax and return to a prone position.

This invigorating exercise brings tone to all the upper body areas. The chest muscles are pulled into play and the excess flesh that develops directly below the neck and rides atop the shoulders, sometimes referred to as a dowager's hump, receives a beneficial massage.

The Waist

Usually where there is a problem of a thickened waist, there are other nearby trouble areas, too. The steady pull of the exercises that melt away rolls of unsightly flesh concealing a perfect waistline can also be effective in toning or paring down the abdomen.

1. Stand erect with the feet slightly apart and the arms hang-

ing loosely by the sides. With the long, slow movements of a robot, bend the body to the left as far as it can comfortably reach, with the left arm reaching as low as possible toward the ankle without bending the knees. Slowly return and continue the bending movement on the right side, reaching downward with the right arm. Without pausing between movements, go from the right to the left and back again, continuing this robot-like movement with a smoothness of body motion.

Twenty times of this exercise twice a day will reduce the most stubborn of out-size waists. If there is any stiffness or difficulty, reduce the number until flexibility is felt.

This next waist whittler will come more easily after some suppleness is gained from the previous exercise. But it can be practiced in easy movements without using any force in conjunction with the first.

2. Standing erect, raise clasped hands above the head. Push the palms upward as far as possible. Take a beauty breath and bring the arms down together on the left side to touch the outer side of the left ankle. Exhale and pause for a moment. Slowly breathe in and return the hands to the position above the head. Repeat the movement by swinging the clasped hands very slowly to the right side of the right ankle.

3. Take a standing position with the feet about twelve inches apart. Extend both arms at shoulder level and begin to beauty breathe. Without bending the knees, twist the body very slowly from the right side to the left, bending at the waist until your right hand is reaching for the left foot. The left arm is extended upward and remains in this position. Hold this pose for a few moments, or as long as there is no strain. Slowly swing back to the original position. Continue to beauty breathe and slowly twist downward with the left hand reaching for the right foot and the right arm extending ceilingward. Hold the position and then slowly return to the original pose.

This slimming and muscle toning action works at the

waistline and abdomen and trims shoulders and arms.

4. Lie flat on the floor in a relaxed position. Beauty breathe in and out. Place your hands beneath your head and support the lower part of the head and the upper part of the neck by interlocking your hands together. Very slowly begin to lift your head and legs simultaneously upward from the floor without bending your knees. After raising them a few inches, slowly return them to the floor.

Repeating this exercise stimulates the abdominal area and helps restore tone and tighten loose skin. Muscles develop resiliency as abdominal fat is worked away.

Here is one of the finest abdominal tighteners. It requires practice to get into the proper position for good effects. But a slow, determined approach to this exercise that will help eliminate sagging abdominal muscles is well worth all the effort required to master it.

5. Lie flat on the floor face up with your arms held comfortably by your sides, palms on the floor. Beauty breathe in and out. With the knees kept straight slowly raise your legs until they are held directly overhead in a vertical position. Use the flattened palms to help reach this position by pushing with them against the floor. Continue to beauty breathe as you push against the floor and slowly raise your legs upward and over your head, aiming for the floor behind your head with your toes. In yoga, this is known as the plough exercise.

This is not always possible the first time one attempts it. Repeated efforts should limber the unused body muscles as the waist is made more flexible and permits the legs to stretch toward the floor. Do not force yourself beyond a comfortable position. Patience in this exercise will help to flatten and tone the abdomen in time.

The Hips

There are many exercises for controlling and tightening the hip area. Sheer indifference is most often responsible for this difficult and frequent figure fault. Lack of physical exercise and careless eating habits are the greatest culprits, but determination and perseverance can really lead to impressive results.

Walking a mile a day helps improve tone and encourage the development of a svelte figure. Bicycling is also one of the best hip exercises. The outdoor type is preferable, but you can create your own indoor yogic bicycling with the use of nothing other than your own legs.

1. Lie flat on the floor face up with the arms by the side. Beauty breathe in and out and create a rhythmic movement of body and breath as you lift the right knee and draw the sole of that foot slowly across the floor. Continue the upward movement of the knee, allowing the foot to leave the floor as you bring the knee as close to the chest as possible. Return the leg to its prone position and at the same time pull back the left leg and allow the foot to slide lightly toward the buttocks as you repeat the movement with this leg. This unified motion should be that of bicycling.

Perform this exercise very slowly. Greater tone comes to the hips from the foot dragging action because the hips are called upon to provide the energy in this exercise. In consequence, the fat is worked away more quickly with this variation of the usual bicycle exercise in which the legs simply pedal in the air.

2. Assume a kneeling position with the buttocks resting on the heels. Place lightly clasped hands in the lap. Extend the hands with the palms turned outward and sit on the right leg. With hands held directly before you as a means of balance, rise upward on the knees and slowly lower yourself, still with arms extended, to sit on your left leg. Repeat several times, or as long as it is comfortable.

This undulating movement works at the hip area and otherwise difficult-to-reach muscles.

3. Lie with the back flat on the floor with your arms spread-eagled to either side on a level with the shoulders and your legs extended before you on the floor. Very slowly raise the

right leg until it is at a right angle to the body. Keep your shoulders on the floor and very slowly without using any force, swing the right leg as close to your left hand as is comfortably possible. Very slowly, return the right leg to an upright position before lowering it carefully to the floor. Inhale going up and exhale coming down.

Raise the left leg overhead and direct it to the right hand before returning it to an upright position and then to the floor. Relax between movements and repeat.

The Thighs

This is another part of the body that can expand very easily. Sedentary people who are occupied in offices, schools and homes soon find that the thighs have begun to spread.

One seldom sees a postman with this condition or anyone involved in a form of work that keeps the body in motion. But chairsitters and housewives are especially susceptible to this unsightly padding. However, the heavy thigh can be avoided if a planned exercise becomes a regular part of the day. If there is no time for walking or other such activity, the following exercise will help you maintain or acquire shapely thighs.

1. Sit erect on the floor with your legs extended straight before you. Slowly draw the knees upward. Slant them in outward and opposite directions until the soles of the feet are touching and the heels are as close to the crotch as is comfortably possible.

Clasp the feet with interlocked hands and very slowly allow the knees to drop toward the floor. Relax and hold this position. Then very slowly and without strain or discomfort, gradually press the knees downward. Hold this position for a moment before allowing the knees to find their own comfortable level.

The inner thighs especially profit from this leg stretching. That area is one of the first to lose tone in a body that isn't sufficiently exercised. By performing this knee-to-floor exercise daily, a tightening process will, in time, trim inches off the thickest thighs.

The Calves

Calves often suffer from insufficient walking. Therefore, special movements are needed if one is to retain or restore a lost curve. In hospital cases of long bed rest, the unused muscles in the calves are the first to deteriorate from enforced inactivity. But exercises which pull directly on poorly toned calves restore both tone and shapeliness.

1. Stand tall on tiptoes with the stomach tucked in, the shoulders held erect and the arms extended straight out in front to provide body balance. Very slowly, beauty breathing in and out and keeping the back straight, allow the knees to bend and lower the buttocks as far down as possible.

Allow the arms to help in controlling your balance by keeping them extended before you. After the buttocks reach the heels, hold this position for several moments, lengthening the time as flexibility increases.

Very slowly, without assistance other than the push of the toes, rise upward to your original position and relax. Repeat as often as is comfortable. If this exercise proves too difficult in the beginning, use the assistance of a heavy chair or table, as support for your hands as you lower yourself toward your heels. You can also place your hands on either side of a doorknob as you gradually bend knees downward. Be sure to have a good grasp and maintain a firm grip.

You can feel the tautening effect on your calves during this exercise. The greater the awareness in the calves, the greater the need for strengthening. However, do not overdo this exercise. Build up to its benefits gradually.

After accomplishing this movement with some ease, repeat the exercise by holding your feet flat on the floor as you lower yourself into a squatting position.

CHAPTER SIXTEEN

Exercises for Trouble Spots

One of the most annoying afflictions women suffer from is that unsightly "lazy-arm" flabbiness so commonly seen, regardless of age. Since men are more physically active than women and seldom have this distressing condition, the only obvious remedy for upper arm flabbiness is exercise.

More diligence is necessary to firm arm muscles than to rid oneself of a bulging abdomen, but the result is just as vital to overall beauty. Special motions are needed to pull at the sagging muscles and restore elasticity.

A woman in her fifties took a job in a local supermarket to help out with heavy family expenses. After several weeks of filling and lifting heavy grocery bags, she noticed a tremendous second benefit to her job. Her upper arms were becoming firm, and folds of loose hanging flesh were tightening up. In time, her arms became as attractive as those of a much younger woman. Without such a job, one can duplicate the effect only by regular exercise.

Upper Arm

1. Stand erect with elbows bent and palms turned upward directly over the shoulders. Imagine that the palms are pushing a heavy box upward until the arms are straight, still with the palms supporting the imaginary box. Without relaxing the tautened arm position, very slowly lower the imagined weight downward to shoulder level again. Repeat.
2. Stand erect with the feet one to two feet apart and the arms extended straight out sideways from the shoulders.

Beauty breathe and push out as far as you can with hands clenched. Very slowly, deliberately not moving the arms, rotate the clenched hands in a complete circle several times. Relax and reverse the circle and repeat.

3. Stand slightly beyond arm's length from a wall. Carefully slant the body forward reaching the arms toward the wall. Press the palms flat against the wall with the arms straight. Beauty breathe and very slowly, bend the arms at the elbows and bring your body close to the wall. Continue to beauty breathe and stiffen your arms as you push yourself away from the wall. Repeat several times a day.

Neck and Throat

Millions of dollars a year are spent on throat creams in an effort to avoid the crepey folds that can appear any year after forty or even earlier.

The reason for them is that layers of supportive fat tucked into the neck and throat area begin to be absorbed with the aging process. Because these fat deposits are not resupplied, the tissue surrounding the disappearing fat is left unsupported. With no internal padding, the skin begins to hang, and without exercise to tighten this area, the throat covering loses tone and sags.

The entire neck and throat area should be treated as one in regaining tone and removing skin folds. This exercise will help keep the head upright and avoid a double chin.

1. Sit or stand upright, with the back straight. Begin to beauty breathe and drop the head toward the chest as far as it will go comfortably. Close the eyes and very slowly direct the head in a circle, from the right side all the way around to center front. Then revolve the head in the other direction.

Keep the shoulders erect and do not move them. Only the head moves in this gentle massaging action to the throat and neck areas. The tendency here is for speed, but only slow movements will work. Allow the head to circle the neck several times, making only one complete turn in either direction in one minute. You may count as your head turns, reaching the count of sixty as your head returns to front and center. After several revolutions in one direction, reverse, and begin from left to right.

Face

Your face reflects your emotions as surely as a clock's face tells the hour. Both reveal the inner movements. Turmoil, fear, hate, greed or anxiety are going to stamp themselves as indelibly on your features as are interest or joy or love.

No amount of skillfully applied makeup can accomplish the effect of a serene countenance. This million-dollar asset has more than one source of origin. If fatigue and tension can't be avoided, they can be helped enormously by a natural diet of unprocessed foods. And physical exercise can utilize good diet and help the body attain the best health possible. If these two habits are established, it is truly a fact that inner and outer serenity become more easily attainable.

Some facial exercises are most helpful in easing tension lines. Since the mouth is the most susceptible to these, we'll begin with that.

The fine lines that create an undesirable sunburst of puckers around the mouth can be effectively dealt with if attacked soon enough. Once they are deeply ingrained, the grooves can be softened by facial exercise and lubricating skin food, but they cannot be easily removed, if at all.

Begin the following lip movements early in your natural beauty plan. Prevention is far better than waiting until trouble appears. Practice the exercises several times a day.

1. Open the mouth to form a small "O." Draw the edges of both lips together as tightly as possible in an attempt to close the "O" without allowing the lips to touch. Visualize a drawstring tightening them. Without relaxing the lips, and without allowing them to form a large "O," attempt to force them open. Relax the mouth and repeat.

Simulating the movements of the hands on a clock with

the facial muscles brings an uplift that affects practically every part of the face. From forehead to chin, the clock-like rotation of both muscle and skin will increase circulation, even as it relaxes.

2. Standing before a mirror and beauty breathing, lift the forehead and follow imaginary clock hands from twelve o'clock around to one, and slowly move the facial muscles in this clockwise direction until you return to the starting point.

Relax and repeat in a counterclockwise direction.

The mouth is actively involved in this exercise, but as you gain more and more control over the facial muscles, you will be able to see a free and easy movement of all areas. Practice both with open and then with closed mouth.

Knees

One can have shapely legs that are beautifully contoured and trim from thigh to ankle, with the exception of a bulge on the inner side of the knee.

Massage is seldom the remedy, for in pounding away at the mass of flesh, one is not really attacking the source of the problem. If the fat accumulation is due to slack muscles in the knee area, the following exercises should be of value.

1. Sitting in a chair, extend both feet, without shoes or stockings, directly before you. Very slowly curl the toes directly under in a tight roll. Hold for a count of ten and release. Now roll the toes upward without moving any other part of the foot, hold for a count of ten and release. Alternate the under curl and the upward roll several times each day.

2. In a standing position, beauty breathe, bend the right knee and raise it toward the chest. Grasp the knee with both hands and draw it in toward the body as close as is comfortably possible. Hold for a count of ten and release. Repeat with the left leg.

Ankles

There is no more effective ankle-slimmer and strengthener than the circular foot roll. While you are sitting or lying down, hold one foot before you and very slowly allow the ankle to inscribe a circle. Be sure you think in terms of the ankle creating the circle rather than the foot, otherwise the ankle may not fully participate. Repeat with the left ankle. And then with both feet at once. Use both clockwise and counterclockwise movements.

CHAPTER SEVENTEEN

Eye Care—Exercises and Wrinkle-Chasers

Far more important than wearing double rows of false eyelashes and creating the perfect arch above the eyes is the care of the eyes themselves.

What is the value of the most carefully blended eyeshadow if the eyes are red-rimmed, fatigued, crisscrossed with red blood veins or squinting in a crinkled view?

For this very important part of your face, daily care must be given in order to protect both health and beauty. A few minutes a day in relaxed exercises can sometimes strengthen weakened eye muscles and help clear up faulty vision. When sight becomes less of a strain, the unattractive squint lines and crow's feet will begin to disappear.

Without additional movement to keep eye muscles elastic, eyestrain can easily develop from unused or slack muscles.

Actually, most of our day we are going against nature's original plan for us. Instead of living outdoors in the natural light, we have moved indoors where we sit under artificial light often concentrating on detailed work.

To counter this artificial over-use of our eyes, a few simple exercises performed daily will greatly reduce the resulting eyestrain, which, if not corrected, leads eventually not only to an abundance of wrinkles, but also to poor vision.

The following eye exercises can easily be performed at one's desk or elsewhere. They offer additional benefits of a "vision break" and one can return, refreshed, to work.

1. A simple method for strengthening eye muscles and removing eye tension requires sitting upright while extending

your right arm directly in front of you. Pointing outward with the index finger, very slowly move it to the right, following the fingertip with the eyes without moving the head. Slowly move the arm as far to the right as your vision will permit before returning it, just as slowly. Using the left arm, repeat the procedure, this time swinging the arm in a straight line to the left.

2. Without moving your head, lift your arm upward to the limit of your vision. Hold this position for a few seconds and slowly drop your arm to the lower vision range. Repeat these exercises several times a day, but work up to this gradually.

3. With eyes wide open, visualize a large-faced clock with the numerals printed just at the edge of your vision. Start with twelve o'clock and very slowly, without moving your head, swing your eyes to one o'clock and on around in a clockwise direction, pausing briefly at each number before moving on to the next one. After returning to twelve o'clock, repeat the exercise counterclockwise, moving the eyes from twelve to eleven, etc.

4. Rolling the head without moving the shoulders is a fine exercise for improved vision. This movement relaxes the eyes and lessens developing wrinkles due to eye strain. Learning to do a loose head roll not only improves the vision by means of increased circulation to the optic nerves, but can relax the entire upper body.

The fresh flow of blood encouraged by the head roll brings needed nourishment to the tissues, and strain eases away with only a few minutes of this movement.

Sitting or standing upright with the spine erect, take a deep breath way down into the abdomen, and very slowly roll the head loosely in a circle that remains comfortable. Do not exaggerate your movements, and if the neck muscles are so tight that your head is confined to a very small circular movement, do not force. Practiced daily, this circle will eventually expand as you limber frozen neck muscles and gain greater suppleness in this region.

Eye Care—Exercises and Wrinkle-Chasers

Try rolling from the right around to the left side, still without moving the shoulders, for two times, and then reverse the procedure. Continue to breathe deeply, in and out, for this is the source of the strength that will send fresh blood coursing to weak and fatigued eyes.

In addition to exercises for toning eye muscles, there are additional helps to control the marring of skin tissue by wrinkles, dark circles and frown lines. Learn to express your thought without grimacing. Many people are inclined to punctuate, describe, or apologize for the contents of their speech by clown-like expressions.

The face should not be used to explain verbal expression. Well-chosen words will convey your meaning, and be more appreciated without distracting facial expressions. Frowns, narrowing of the eyes and other manifestations of uncertainty do not present either a pretty or helpful picture. Use adequate speech and save your face.

Of course this is not to say one should not have any expression at all. But these expressions should be relaxed, and show the more pleasant aspects of one's personality. Laugh lines seldom seem to distress their owners as much as frown lines or wrinkles caused by squinting or habitually downturned lips. Laugh lines add animation to the face.

However, the quick-to-laugh personality often pays for charm with crinkle lines around the eyes.

Crow's feet are never pretty and can spoil even the most carefully made-up face. But daily loving attention given this area will bring untold rewards. Honey, our old friend, helps mightily in delaying the formation of these depth lines. For tightening up the skin around the eyes, mix a teaspoon of honey with one egg white. Blend together well and pat the mixture into the tissue around the eyes.

Gently stretch the lines apart, not by pulling, but rather by trying to return the un-elastic skin to its former position before the wrinkles came. Allow the mixture to dry before removing it with tepid water. Apply a cream to the area afterward and pat it in thoroughly, right up to the eye lines, without, of course, getting it into the eyes. The under-eye area has a minimum of oil glands, and whenever an astringent type of beauty aid is used, the drying effects must be countered by a rich cream.

Many women complain of baggy, puffy, or dark-circled eyes. Some old recipes for these problems are just as effective now as they ever were.

1. The darkened areas beneath the eyes usually respond well to a potato compress. After several applications, the unsightly black-eye will be much lightened by mineral-rich, organically grown potatoes.

Grate a small, scrubbed potato and gather enough to fill two small gauze squares. Lie down and apply this to the darkened areas and remain in a prone position, relaxed, for half an hour. Sponge off and pat in a few drops of salad or nut oil.

2. Use grated cucumber in the gauze squares and proceed as with the grated potato.

3. To reduce puffiness directly under the eye, common table salt, preferably sea salt, will sometimes do the trick. Dip small cotton pads into a solution of one cup of hot water into which a teaspoon of salt has been thoroughly dissolved. Lie down and apply the pads directly over the puffy area. Allow them to remain on until they cool and then rinse the area with cool water and blot dry.

4. Tea packs also work marvels on puffy eyes. Steep two bags in boiling water for a few minutes and while they are still warm—not hot—place them directly over the eyes while you are lying down. Relax for fifteen minutes, rinse and apply any salad oil to the area.

5. The herb eyebright has relieved red-streaked eyes for many centuries. Eyestrain in previous times was promptly treated by preparing an astringent lotion of the lovely herb that even today forms the basis for commercial eyewashes. According to the Doctrine of Signatures, the interesting but little known medieval belief that says each plant meant for

medicinal use has its purpose written somewhere on its leaves, stem or flower, the lovely eyebright is well named. A yellow eye is emblazoned upon its small purple-tinged white blossom.

Prepare your own eye lotion by pouring a cup of boiling water over one teaspoon of the dried herb and steeping it until it cools. Strain and bathe the eyes in this soothing liquid whenever they are tired, sting from dust or just need refreshing.

CHAPTER EIGHTEEN

Perfumes, Scents and Potpourris

According to legend, the goddess Venus was the first female to use perfume. She created her beauty and charisma from her Olympian store of carefully guarded secrets. But through an indiscretion on the part of one of her nymphs, Venus's methods of obtaining the fragrances of garden, wood and field were disclosed to mortal man.

It was through these secrets that Paris, Helen of Troy's lover, was able to supply her with the means to acquire the beauty that launched the thousand ships.

No matter how the art of extracting the lovely scents from flowers, spices and perfumed woods—sources of the ingredients for natural perfumes—came to us, it has been an exotic and fascinating heritage.

Knowledge about the effects of perfumes and other scenting mediums can greatly increase one's pleasure and personal charm.

It is considered essential to find one's own scent; *your* essence that will linger in someone's memory, or surround you with mystery, intrigue and delight.

In a perfume shop in Paris, on the rue Caumartin, the *parfumeuse* will not sell a perfume which seems to contradict a woman's appearance or personality. For example, one diminutive woman requested a heavy-scented, overpoweringly seductive perfume. Reluctantly the chemist rubbed a bit onto the woman's underwrist area and waited for the alcohol to evaporate. After the scent was warmed by the woman's body heat, the *parfumeuse* sniffed the wrist with distaste.

"Not for you, Madame," she said. "You are not the sexy type, the siren or the sultry. Instead, just as I thought, your perfume must be selected from flower scents—light, airy and sweet."

The purchaser at first seemed disappointed, but as she sampled the scents offered her, she found one that pleased her and left the shop feeling that she had learned a valuable lesson.

While we may choose to think of ourselves as one kind of personality, we may unconsciously be imitating someone else. Again, it is far better to study oneself and carefully choose a suitable scent.

There have always been costly oils imported from exotic parts of the world. The perfume industry of southern France is noted for its use of fresh flowers, barks, herbs and resins, even though synthetics are also used nowadays.

But there are many delightful scents to be made simply by gathering the necessary ingredients from the garden. Producing your own toilet waters and perfumes becomes a fascinating pastime.

Attar of Roses

The beautiful flower from which attar of roses, a fragrant oil, is made is surely the queen of all flowers, and the rose blossom with its delightful scent has played a crowning role in myth and history.

Flora found the body of a beautiful nymph, a daughter of the dryads and, together with Venus and the Graces, transformed it into the rose. Apollo blessed the new flower with his beams and Bacchus appeared with nectar and Vertumnus with perfume. Pomona wafted her fruit over the young branches while Flora crowned them with a diadem prepared by the Celestials to create the queen of flowers.

Whatever the beginning of the rose, its delights have long been incorporated into pleasant living. Pliny says Roman food was either covered with rose petals or sprinkled with rose perfume. Romans also extracted the juice of the rose for use in body unguents. After the liquid was removed, the petals were dried and powdered to use on the body as a deodorant.

Centuries after the Romans anointed their bodies with rose creams, a Grand Mogul of Persia extravagantly ordered his garden canals filled with rose water. His princess noticed a sweetly scented scum floating on the water and had it collected. She and the women of her court treasured this perfumed mass, and so it was that attar of roses was introduced to the world.

If you have a rose garden, it is perfectly possible to make attar of roses. Locate a glazed earthenware jar and fill it with rose petals separated from the stem. Pour spring or purified water over them to cover and place the jar in direct sunlight for three or four days. Bring the jar in each night and return it to the sun each day. Check the contents daily and on the third or fourth day, you should see small globules of yellow oil floating on the surface. At the end of a week, a thin scum should cover the water. This strange mass will be the fabulous attar of roses, and in monetary value it is worth practically its weight in gold.

Use cotton squares tied to a stick to dip into the covering and absorb this precious oil. Squeeze out the oil into a waiting phial or small glass jar. An eye dropper could be used. But be careful not to extend the tip of the dropper into the water beneath the layer of oil.

Attar of roses sells for one hundred dollars an ounce. What do you do with it? Make your own scented rose water, such as used to come in deep blue bottles printed with pastel paintings. Or use it to scent cosmetics.

Another method of extracting the exquisite oil of roses is with the use of olive or almond oil. Place dried rose petals in a glass pot and cover with the finest grade of oil, whether olive or almond. Simmer over a very low heat until the oil has fully extracted the color of the roses and their perfume.

A more complicated method of gaining the essence of rose perfume requires placing a layer of dried rose petals in an empty jar, sprinkling fine salt over them and covering this with a layer of soft, absorbent cotton which has been dipped into the finest grade of oil. Continue the layering procedure until the jar is filled. Now place a lid over the top and put into the sun. Oil will develop anywhere from ten days to three weeks. Squeeze out the oil when it appears and place in a glass jar or phial.

Potpourri

Once you have discovered the delight of making your own potpourri, you will never give it up. These scented mixtures can be perpetuated for years with the proper attention. However, they are so easy to prepare that it is an actual pleasure to renew them yearly, changing the fragrance with each season's offerings of pungent or airy scents.

Any scented flower can be used, but the ones producing the loveliest effects are roses, lavender, lily of the valley, narcissus blossoms, orange blossoms, violets, carnations and lilac.

The flowers to be used should be gathered in the morning just after the sun has dried the dew from the petals. Some people prefer to gather them earlier and spread the petals on an outdoor table in the shade until the dew has dried.

After the petals are dry, toss them into a large basket or other shallow container, and each day repeat the procedure until you have enough flower petals to fill a selected jar which has a lid or cover. A two-quart soup tureen is an excellent container. When the petals are fully dry, place them in layers in their container and sprinkle a layer of sea salt between them.

Now place the lid on the jar or bowl, and once each day for a week stir up the contents from the bottom of the jar. For a spiced scent, at the end of the week, add three ounces of allspice to the jar's mixture. Repeat the stirring process for three more days, each day adding one-fourth ounce each of whole allspice and cracked cinnamon sticks.

At the end of the three days, add one ounce each of the following coarsely ground spices: cinnamon, cloves, mace, allspice, nutmeg, lemon peel and orange peel. Allow the container to remain closed for one month, after which time it may be opened for a few minutes whenever you want to perfume a room with the delightful fragrance. Always replace the lid tightly and occasionally stir up the contents.

LAVENDER SACHET

½ pound lavender flowers
½ ounce dried mint
½ ounce dried thyme
¼ ounce ground caraway
¼ ounce ground cloves
1 ounce sea salt

Detach the lavender flowers and leaves from their stems. Mix all the ingredients together and place in small silk or cambric bags. Scatter in chests of drawers or closets or pin directly onto clothing in the closet for fragrance.

SANDALWOOD POWDER SACHET

¼ pound Tonka beans
1 pound dried rose petals
1 pound orris root
¼ pound sandalwood (also called santalum)
¼ pound dried lemon verbena leaves
¼ teaspoon oil of rose

Grind all the dry ingredients together into a powder and sprinkle in the oil of rose. Blend together well and apportion into small bags having a drawstring. Or place an amount in the middle of a handkerchief or cotton square, gather the ends together and tie with a pretty ribbon.

The same method is used for the following sachets.

LEMON SACHET

1 pound dried lemon peel
4 ounces lemon geranium leaves
1 ounce oil of bergamot
3 teaspoons oil of lemon
½ teaspoon balm

ROSE SACHET

1 ounce orris root
8 ounces rose petals
8 ounces lavender flowers
1 ounce coriander seed
1 ounce cloves
1 ounce whole cinnamon

Perfumes, Scents and Potpourris

LAVENDER-MINT SACHET

½ ounce any kind of mint   ¼ ounce coriander seeds
½ pound lavender flowers   ¼ ounce whole cinnamon

Lavender water brings to mind handmade lace curtains, velvet chairs and sprigged muslin gowns. This perfumed water was used to scent cambric handkerchiefs that were gently waved about one's face on a warm summer's day. Bits of cotton, soaked in lavender water, were tucked into undergarments and dropped into reticules. And wherever a lady went, she left behind her a faint but delightful freshness.

One of the easiest ways to prepare lavender toilet water is to buy oil of lavender. This is, of course, simpler than distilling one's own, and if you have the small bottle of essential oil on hand, it requires little effort to shake up a bottle of toilet water whenever it is desired.

LAVENDER TOILET WATER

1 quart ethyl alcohol   ½ ounce oil of lavender

Mix the oil of lavender with a little alcohol and dissolve well. Add the remaining alcohol in a thin stream, beating well all the while. Pour into glass jars and seal with rubber rings. Allow this to mature for two months before using. Shake the containers frequently during this time to insure blending.

Variations of the plain lavender water offer endless sources of delightful toilet waters. After experimenting with a few of the following combinations you can develop your own scent.

PRINCESS LAVENDER WATER

3 teaspoons oil of lavender   1 ounce rose water
½ ounce oil of cloves   6 ounces ethyl alcohol

Mix the oil of lavender and cloves with a little alcohol; dissolve well. Add the remaining alcohol in a thin stream and continue beating. Stir in the rose water and proceed as in the previous recipe.

FLORIDA WATER

1 ounce oil of bergamot ½ teaspoon oil of cinnamon
½ ounce tincture of benzoin

Place the three ingredients into a two-quart glass jar and cover with one quart of ethyl alcohol. Allow to stand for a month, shaking frequently during that time. Filter through filter paper and pour into a well-stoppered bottle.

BALSAM OF A THOUSAND FLOWERS

¼ ounce essence of cloves ¼ ounce thyme
¼ ounce balsam of Peru ¼ pint orange flower water
½ ounce bergamot 1 quart ethyl alcohol
¼ ounce orange oil

Place all the scents together in a two-quart glass container with a lid. Pour the alcohol slowly over the ingredients, stirring constantly to produce a complete blending. Let the mixture stand for ten days before filtering and bottling for use.

VIOLET WATER

1 pound powdered orris root 1 pint ethyl alcohol

Mix the orris root and alcohol together thoroughly by placing in a lidded jar and shaking well. Allow this to stand on the dregs for ten days before filtering through filter paper to remove the orris root.

ROSE WATER

½ teaspoon attar of roses 1 pint ethyl alcohol

Dissolve the rose oil in carefully warmed alcohol. While still warm, place in a two-gallon jug and add one and three-fourths gallons of distilled water, heated to about 190 degrees. Cork the jug and shake, cautiously at first, and then more vigorously, until the contents are cold. A note of caution: warm the alcohol by placing the opened container in a pan of hot water, away from the fire.

Another method of producing rose water requires twelve

drops of attar of roses placed on a half ounce of cube sugar. Add to this one teaspoon of carbonate of magnesia. Put this into a fruit jar and slowly pour in one quart of distilled or soft water, stirring well. To this, add two ounces of ethyl alcohol. Pour this over filtering paper which has been placed over a second jar. The filtering paper removes the magnesia.

Lovely scents, referred to as tinctures, are easily obtained by using the fresh blossoms from a flower garden. The tinctures are delightful to use on clothing, linens or as a personal scent when placed on balls of cotton and tucked into one's clothing.

Any strongly-scented flower can be used, such as the jonquil in the springtime, the hyacinth, violet, jasmine or honeysuckle.

Pack the selected flowers, either of one scent, or a combination, into a fruit jar and cover the blossoms with alcohol. Allow these to steep for several days and then strain the liquid through a fine cloth. Catch the flowers in the cloth and squeeze out the remaining essence. Now add fresh flowers to this liquid and repeat the procedure until you have the strength of scent you wish.

GERANIUM PERFUME

Using the same method as with flowers, pack the sweet-smelling green leaves of the rose geranium—or other scented geranium—into a glass jar and fill it with alcohol. Allow this to stand for a few weeks before straining and bottling for use. These leaves, too, may be replaced from time to time during the steeping process.

COLOGNE WATER

1 pint ethyl alcohol
1 teaspoon oil of lavender
1 teaspoon bergamot
1 teaspoon essence of lemon
1 teaspoon orange water

Mix all the oils and essence together and slowly stir in the alcohol, beating all the while. Place in corked bottles and allow to mellow for two months.

Sources of Ingredients

Ingredients available at pharmacies:

Almond oils
Benzoin
Camphor and camphorated oil
Castor oil
Cocoa butter
Cod liver oil
Complexion brush
Ethyl alcohol
Fuller's earth
Gum arabic
Henna leaves
Hydrous lanolin
Perfumed oils
Talcum, unscented
Witch hazel

Ingredients available at health food stores:

Acerola berries
Almond butter and paste
Eyebright
Herbal teas such as camomile, coltsfoot, elder flower, papaya-mint, etc.
Natural foods such as whole grains—oats, barley, wheat germ and grain-grown brewer's yeast, whole-grain flours
Natural vitamins
Organically grown nuts
Sea salt

Sources of Ingredients

Seeds to sprout such as alfalfa,
   mung, soy, etc.
Seed sprouters
Unrefined (cold pressed) oils
Vegetable soaps
Yogurt makers

Other sources:

Beeswax—Hobby and art shops, beekeepers, and Caswell-Massey, Co., Ltd., 114 East 25th St., New York, N.Y. 10010.

Comfrey plants—North Central Comfrey Producers, Box 195B, Glidden, Wis. 54527

Dishcloth gourds—George W. Park Co., Greenwood, S.C. 29646

Friction Gloves—J.D. Browne, Ghirardelli Sq., 900 North Pt., San Francisco, Calif. 98904

Potpourri, dried—Capriland Herb Farm, Silver St., Coventry, Conn. 06238 and Caswell-Massey, Ltd.

Most herbs, oils, flowers, plant dyes, waxes, etc., can be found at the Indiana Botanic Gardens, Hammond, Ind., or other botanical supply houses.

Glossary

Almond meal—the finely ground nutmeats from the almond tree used for pore cleansing and refining.

Almond oil—extracted from the almond nutmeats and used for centuries as a soothing oil for the entire body.

Aloe vera—expressed juice from the leaves of this spike-toothed plant has been found to have healing qualities promotive of good skin health.

Apple cider vinegar—fermented apple cider producing an acid liquid useful when mixed with water in restoring the natural acid mantle to the skin.

Apricot oil—extracted oil from the apricot kernel, rich in polyunsaturated fatty acids.

Attar of roses—costly oil requiring four thousand pounds of rose petals to produce one pound of oil.

Balm—a fragrant herb, also called Melissa, containing an oil of lemon fragrance used in making perfumes.

Balsam of Tolu—resin from tropical balsamic trees producing a delicate hyacinth-like fragrance.

Barley—a cereal of nutritious content which, when cooked, produces a milky fluid soothing to irritated skin.

Benzoin—balsamic resin from trees growing in Sumatra and Java.

Bergamot—essential oil extracted from the rind of the pear-shaped orange.

Bran—the nutritious outer covering of grain, removed during the milling process, but possessing valuable nutrients.

Brewer's yeast—a superior source of protein and B vitamins.

Camomile—a fragrant herb used for the golden flowers containing a cleansing oil with bleaching properties.

Cocoa butter—solidified oil from the roasted cacao bean. Excellent for dry skins.

Comfrey—a plant with mucilaginous leaves which soothe and heal the skin and body.

Curd soap—soap containing milk.

Cuttlefish—a marine mollusk; its finely powdered shell produces an abrasive.

Elder flowers—blossoms which produce a pleasantly scented and soothing lotion. All parts of the plant are used in various lotions and creams, but the blossoms have long been considered useful in cosmetics because of their soothing and refreshing qualities.

Ethyl alcohol—used in cosmetic formulas and as an aid in dissolving perfume oils.

Fuller's earth—claylike earthy substance rich in minerals. Effectively used in facial masques because of its stimulating effect.

Frankincense—a fragrant gum coming from resinous trees in East Africa. Used as a fixative in Oriental perfumes.

Gum arabic—a composition of magnesium, calcium and potassium salts of arabic acid. Prized as a thickener and stabilizer, among other uses. It has also been used as a food even though its nutritious content is slight.

Gum benzoin—balsamic resin in solid form.

Lanolin—fatty substance coming from the wool of sheep. Much favored for use in fine cosmetics because in composition it closely resembles the fat in the human body and therefore is easily absorbed when placed on the skin.

Lobelia—also called Indian tobacco, the leaves and roots are used externally in treatment of skin ailments.

Malt extract—germinated grain, usually barley.

Neat's-foot oil—a pale yellow oil coming from the shinbones and feet of cattle.

Orange water—a delicately fragrant liquid produced from distillation of orange blossoms.

Orris root—the dried root of the scented iris. Used in making perfumes and sachets.

Potpourri—a mixture of dried flowers kept in a jar and used to perfume a room.

Purified water—filtered water.

Rosemary—an evergreen herb of modern and ancient usage in both cosmetics and cooking. Especially valued for its pungent essential oil for skin and hair.

Rose hips—the small red berry on wild rose bushes used as a valuable source of vitamin C.

Rose water—scented water produced by distilling, or other method, rose petals or rose oil with water.

Sesame seed oil—oil from the tiny sesame seeds which has excellent keeping qualities. Its nutritious content contributes to its value as both an internal and external food.

Soapbark chips—the bark of an American shrub which serves as a soap substitute.

Stinging nettle—herb that grows wild, with formic acid in its leaves which blisters the skin on contact. Must be handled with great care. Helpful as a stimulating hair wash if used with great caution.

Southernwood—lemon-scented herb with astringent qualities.

Spermaceti—a white, odorless wax derived from the sperm oil of whales. Useful in cosmetic preparations.

Sandalwood—fragrant wood from East Indian trees and used in sachets and potpourris.

Storax—a scented balsamic resin.

Sage—a strongly scented herb beneficially used in shampoos, rinses and as a tea.

Sea salt—if coming directly from evaporated sea water, sea salt contains at least thirty trace elements, including calcium and magnesium.

Tincture of benzoin—liquid form of benzoin.

Tonka beans—seed of a tropical American tree which in scent is strongly suggestive of vanilla.

Wheat germ—a valuable source of vitamin E, coming from the heart of the wheat plant which is removed during refining.

Witch hazel—fluid extract from the shrub which offers refreshing and invigorating qualities.